Agricultural Development and Nutrition

Agricultural Development and Nutrition

Edited by Arnold Pacey
and Philip Payne

HUTCHINSON
London Melbourne Sydney Auckland Johannesburg
WESTVIEW PRESS
Boulder, Colorado

by arrangement with
the Food and Agriculture Organization of the United Nations and
the United Nations Children's Fund

Hutchinson and Co. (Publishers) Ltd
An imprint of the Hutchinson Publishing Group
17–21 Conway Street, London W1P 6JD

Hutchinson Publishing Group (Australia) Pty Ltd
16–22 Church Street, Hawthorn, Melbourne, Victoria 3122

Hutchinson Group (NZ) Ltd
32–34 View Road, PO Box 40–086, Glenfield, Auckland 10

Hutchinson Group (SA) (Pty) Ltd
PO Box 337, Bergvlei 2012, South Africa

First published 1985

Published in 1985 in the United States of America by
  Westview Press, Inc.
  5500 Central Avenue
  Boulder, Colorado 80301
  Frederick A. Praeger, President and Publisher

Set in Linotype Times by Saxon Ltd, Derby, England.

Printed and bound in Great Britain by
Anchor Brendon Ltd, Tiptree, Essex.

British Library Cataloguing in Publication Data

Agricultural development and nutrition.
  1. Food crops—Tropics
  I. Pacey, Arnold   II. Payne, Philip
  338.1'9'0913   SB176.T7
Library of Congress Catalog Card Number 85-50544
ISBN (UK) 0 09 161330 2 cased
     (UK) 0 09 161331 0 paper
     (US) 0-8133-0265-X cased

Contents

action is to use an analytical framework which is itself action-oriented. 'Functional classification' is such a framework. It provides descriptions of population groups which made administrative sense, and which enable agriculture, nutrition and health policies to be better targeted on situations which give rise to malnutrition. Examples of the implication for some interventions are discussed.

Foreword

During the decade which followed the World Food Conference held in l974 in Rome, much debate, research and evaluation has focused on the impact of development strategies on the prevalence of malnutrition. Within the UN system the Food and Agriculture Organization (FAO) and the Children's Fund (UNICEF) have been actively involved in promoting new approaches in this field. FAO has been at the forefront of recent efforts to improve the nutritional impact of agriculture and rural development. UNICEF's well-known work guides and supports many types of development that relate to child welfare and services, including the problems of access to food and feeding of children.

There is a unanimity of opinion in all circles that the agriculture sector lies at the centre of any solution to the world's food problems. Yet the sobering thought that has become all too evident in recent years is that food production alone is not the answer. Rapid progress in production and exports of food commodities are found to co-exist with malnutrition even in the same areas of certain countries. Therefore while increased food production is an essential precondition, improved distribution is also necessary to overcome inadequate food consumption and malnutrition. The work that remains to be done is the application of suitable approaches through which agriculture and rural development can prevent the waste of human resources and potential which is caused by malnutrition.

This text, prepared by the Nutrition Policy Unit of the London School of Hygiene and Tropical Medicine, is an exposé of the many food consumption-related problems which need to be considered alongside agricultural production issues in development. It examines those social, environmental, economic and political factors that determine the degree to which people have access to food and can assimilate its nutrients. After reviewing the present scientific knowledge of energy, nutrient requirements and human growth, the authors concentrate on the many obstacles rural families face in trying to satisfy their basic food needs.

They argue for a balanced agricultural and rural development which would alleviate not only the technical constraints to increased production but also those many social, economic and political impediments that prevent people from having access to the foods that are produced.

This compilation of materials originally prepared for a UNICEF/FAO/Indian Council of Agricultural Research Workshop, is therefore a most important contribution to the thinking that has evolved recently about an interdisciplinary approach to food and nutrition problems. It will stimulate agriculturalists, rural development experts, food and nutrition planners and nutritionists all over the world in devising development strategies that are as concerned about impact as they are about outputs.

FAO and UNICEF are pleased to have supported the preparation of this manuscript and, while not necessarily endorsing its every argument, are gratified to be associated with a book which provides a modern and responsible vision of the basic themes and questions which they consider must guide development. The text is intended to stimulate interdisciplinary thought, discussion, research and action at the village, district, national and international level. By questioning the weaknesses of present approaches it cannot help but challenge all of us to search for more effective answers to food and nutrition problems in future development.

Preface

Starting in 1971, the Government of India, with the assistance of FAO, UNICEF and UNDP, embarked on a long-term programme to extend and reinforce the subject of human nutrition in higher education. The programme envisaged the teaching of food and nutrition subjects in agricultural, veterinary and home science colleges, and these institutions have been assisted in building up food and nutrition departments to undertake training and research in subjects related to nutrition.

Since 1980, under the title 'Education in Food and Nutrition in Agricultural Universities' (EFNAG) the programme has developed both in direction and content.

The general objective remains the same: to improve the nutrition of rural families and the means of achieving this is through three main aims:

1. to introduce a wider understanding of nutritional issues in the agricultural sector in order to incorporate nutritional considerations in agricultural programmes and hence bring about better nutrition;
2. to promote an understanding of the factors contributing to malnutrition, especially those related to poverty, with special reference to infant malnutrition;
3. to develop a more comprehensive view of training in agriculture and allied subjects that includes elements of food and nutrition education and basic services for children: this broader view should encompass the human aspects of agriculture, such as

development communication, extension methods, programme planning and food planning.

Of particular concern has been the need to strengthen the capacities of agricultural universities to include a nutrition dimension into the training of post-graduate students, and to lay the foundations of an expanding programme of applied and operational research in areas which link the production of food with the nutrition of rural people.

As an expression of that concern, the Indian Council of Agricultural Research, with the sponsorship of FAO and UNICEF, organised a workshop at Haryana Agricultural University in April 1982. The Nutrition Policy Unit of the London School of Hygiene and Tropical Medicine was invited to propose a programme of topic areas; to provide background working papers for the review sessions; and to conduct and co-ordinate the proceedings generally.

The objective of the workshop was to review in depth those aspects of the science of food and nutrition which are relevant to agriculture and to rural development, and similarly those aspects of agricultural change which have a direct or indirect impact on the nutritional condition of human populations. With this review as a background, the workshop was then to determine priorities for the inclusion of nutrition topics into programmes of post-graduate training in agriculture and home science, and hence to provide guidelines for future curriculum and research programme development. This book has been based for the main part on material presented to the workshop, and on a record of the discussions which ensued.

It is conventional to preface books of this kind with broad statements about the critical importance of improving the nutritional conditions of human populations, and of accepting that such improvement should be an explicit objective of development. It is logical to assume that the pace and direction of agricultural change will be a critical factor in achieving this objective: more people consuming a better diet must have implications for food production, and more effective deployment of the means of production should be reflected in more people able to afford to eat adequately.

However, having indicated this fundamental relationship, it has usually been assumed that the objective of improving the nutrition of human populations at the same time as improving the practice of agriculture will be achieved automatically through bringing about an interchange between the two academic disciplines of nutrition and of agriculture. But what exactly should be the nature of that exchange? Should it be factual knowledge? Will malnutrition be reduced if agricultural students in future know that there are 10 amino acids essential for health, or that beans contain more protein than rice, or that vitamin A deficiency can be prevented by eating green vegetables? Or should the exchanges be of concepts, of the nature of the processes, social and economic, as well as physiological, which result in malnourished individuals?

We believe that it is particularly important at this time to take a critical look at how the two disciplines, agriculture and nutrition, should be expected to interact. We hope that this will be especially fruitful in the context of post-graduate activities, since this is traditionally the area in which subjects develop and new concepts are formed. Not the least reason for the timeliness is that despite the widely acknowledged importance of adequate nutrition as a basic component of human welfare, and despite the manifest success of agriculture in supporting the growing populations of the world, malnutrition persists. We have both more food *and* more destitute and hungry people. How can the connection be made between our growing technical capacity to generate wealth from the soil on the one hand and our understanding of the biological and social needs of man for food on the other? One thing is certain, there are no easy answers, and the reader of this book will search in vain for prescriptions, progress will come only through the realisation that the real problems and solutions lie in the nature of social and political institutions and the human relationships that underlie them. For some people this realisation is painful, and leads either to a rejection of science as irrelevant, or to a retreat into the more comfortable distractions of academic research. We shall be happy if this book helps to strengthen the view that curiosity about the way the world works, and the urge to extend knowledge about what things are possible in the world through analysis and criticism can be applied to the solution of the problems that give rise to hunger.

Peter Cutler
Elizabeth Dowler
Barbara Harriss
Philip Payne
Erica Wheeler

Those whose names appear above are the members of the Nutrition Policy Unit of the Department of Human Nutrition at the London School of Hygiene and Tropical Medicine. All of them contributed material to the book. It could not have been written, though, without the help of many other people, in particular N.S. Jodha, Claire Kelly, David Nabarro, Adam Pain, Paul Richards, John Rivers, Young Ok Seo and Anne Thomson, who either work with us, or generously allowed us to use their work. We are also grateful to Madeleine Green and Barbara Kenmir who typed the manuscript.

Above all the book is the result of the integrating perspectives and unstinting labour of Arnold Pacey.

Our grateful thanks go to Margaret Khalakdvia and her staff at Haryana Agricultural University, and to Franciso Coloane of UNICEF for their outstanding hospitality, constant encouragement and careful arrangements which ensured the smooth running of the workshop.

The costs of editing and preparation of the manuscript were borne by FAO and UNICEF. However, neither of these organisations are responsible for any of the views or opinions expressed herein.

Philip Payne

PART ONE

Limits to Measurement

'The people are crying out for bread and we are going to give them statistics.'

John Boyd-Orr in 1945 on proposed terms of reference for FAO (see Orr 1966, pp. 20, 162)

1 Food systems and needs*

Changed perspectives

During the last three decades, the application of nutritional science to the problems of hunger and malnutrition has passed through a phase of great confidence and hope, followed by one of increasing uncertainty and doubt. Twenty years ago, a book such as this would have discussed well-defined nutritional interventions, aimed at achieving some equally well-defined nutritional objectives. Very little space would have been devoted to questioning the validity of those objectives, or the effectiveness of the programmes themselves. In so far as progress towards reducing malnutrition was acknowledged to be slight, this would have been interpreted as showing the need for more extended programmes, hence for more resources, and especially for more trained people to be deployed.

The connection between nutrition and agriculture would have been presumed to rest on a number of premises: that hunger would be eliminated if there were an increase in the overall production of food; that malnutrition is often caused by deficiencies of specific nutrients (e.g. protein) and that this can best be countered by emphasis on the production of certain kinds of foods, or by fortification or enrichment of staples; that poor

---

*This chapter is based mainly on material prepared by Philip Payne; see Rivers and Payne (1982) and Payne (1982).

nutrition is often the result simply of ignorance; and hence there is a general need to educate people on how to make proper use of the resources available to them. Infectious disease, though recognised to interact with malnutrition, would be regarded as essentially a separate problem to be dealt with by specifically designed programmes.

There has been a fairly radical change of viewpoint over the last two decades. This has been broadly for three reasons. Firstly, there has been a change in concept: malnutrition, previously regarded as something caused by single physical factors, is now accepted as having multiple causes, many of which are closely linked to the conditions of inequality of resources, or poverty, and of social discrimination. Changes in the system of food production which leave these conditions unchanged will also leave malnutrition unchanged or may even aggravate it. Indeed, we have witnessed some countries becoming net exporters of food, while sections of their populations remain inadequately fed, or even experience famine. In addition to this, among young children especially, malnutrition is so intimately related to infectious disease that it makes no practical sense to pursue programmes aimed at improving food consumption without also tackling at least some of the environmental causes of such disease. This may lead the nutritionist to encourage improvements in water supply, sanitation, housing and domestic fuel.

The second reason for a changed perspective is that there has been progress in our understanding of the physiological and biochemical processes underlying malnutrition. We now know that man has the capacity to adapt to a fairly wide range of dietary situations, and that only when that adaptive capacity is stretched beyond its limits does the body fail to maintain its functional capacity,* and malnutrition ensues.

Thirdly, there is a growing awareness that many of the more

---

*Functional capacity here is taken to mean all aspects of the behaviour of an individual in response to the environment, such as physical and mental activity, response to stress, disease etc. This should not be confused with the term 'functional classification' which is used in later chapters.

conventional types of nutrition programme have not achieved what was hoped of them. Interventions such as the promotion of high-protein crops, food delivery systems aimed at young children, and projects for educating people about the nutritional value of foods, have often been totally ineffective, or effective only as short-term palliatives. Frequently they have also distracted attention from the need to attack more fundamental problems.

It is in this context of doubts and questioning about past ideas that we need to review the relationship between knowledge of nutrition and planning for agriculture. We believe that from a basis of analysis and criticism, we shall be able to begin a synthesis. But the ideas that will carry us forward will be different from those of the past. They will include ideas about food systems, about the epidemiology of malnutrition, and about 'livelihoods'. They will also include suggestions about the use of indicators, and ways of understanding the multiple causes of illness and deprivation. These and other concepts give us a new point of departure, so that we should not expect simply to substitute a new set of nutrition programmes, more potent and more efficient than the old – a set of 'right' answers to substitute for the 'wrong' ones. There are no simple answers, and whatever it is that a nutritional approach to human problems can provide, it is not likely to give us any short-cut solutions or technical fixes. The problems of malnutrition will be overcome as and when we overcome those of poverty, deprivation and disease. But we are all concerned with these, and therefore we could well begin by asking: what is so special about the nutritional viewpoint? Why should we be especially sensitive about nutritional needs rather than economic or social needs?

One clear lesson from the past is that when a particular problem at first sight requires nutritional expertise for its solution, this analysis is not always borne out by closer critical analysis. The skill and integrity of a profession rest at least as much on its willingness to show when it cannot and should not play a key role, as on its ability to demonstrate the effectiveness of its methods when they are relevant. However, there is a general case for concerning ourselves with nutrition and with food as a fundamental aspect of agricultural development, and this rests on two propositions.

The first identifies the nutritional status of a person as both the outcome of the process of acquiring, consuming and utilising food, and one of the critical inputs to that process: the food a woman or a man eats decides the amount of effort she or he can afford to invest in order to secure food in the future. If we can measure nutritional status, therefore, we have a unique index of the impact upon individuals of the whole system of production, utilisation and exchange.

The other proposition is related to this: it is that, of all the symbols and objects of social exchange, food is arguably the most basic. Co-operation in the acquisition of food, and its sharing among the members of a family marked the beginning of the social evolution of mankind. The extent of an individual's integration with society can be measured by the adequacy and security of his or her ability to produce, control, purchase, borrow or otherwise acquire food (i.e. his 'food entitlement' (Sen, 1981)).*

This book is focused on a range of topics which impinge upon different stages and processes operating within the food 'system'; that is to say, the system comprising the production, distribution, consumption and biological utilisation of food. Figure 1.1 shows, in a much simplified way, a few of the key relationships and processes which will be discussed. It is not intended as a complete definition of the 'system', but more a starting framework within which we may wish to elaborate certain areas. Then, by understanding *how* people become malnourished in terms of processes within the system, we may be better able to make statements about *who* such people are, and to describe their relationship with production and the basis of their entitlement to food. Malnutrition, in this context, is a symptom or signal that certain processes are regularly occurring in the lives of people which, if disregarded, will result in the continued generation of sickness and physiological impairment.

---

*Full references quoted in the text are contained in the Bibliography beginning on p.220.

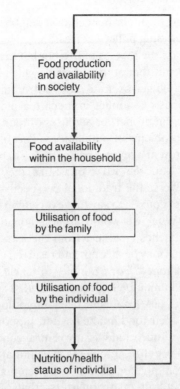

Figure 1.1　The food system as it is envisaged in this book, in its simplest form

Analysis of the nutritional problems within a society may therefore have implications for agriculture at many different levels. At one level, it may consider the impact of agricultural change on the ability of people to earn an entitlement to food. To produce more, but at a cost many people cannot afford, may be self-defeating. An orientation of technology to production, which neglects problems of consumption, needs to be corrected. At other levels, the analysis points to the need for an integrated approach by planners to the development of land resources for food, for fuel and for cash crops. It underlines the need to improve the domestic environment as well as to plan resource inputs to agriculture. It may also indicate the need to avoid certain directions of change because of the danger of aggravating the risk of malnutrition, or may at least demonstrate the cost of that effect in assessing policy choices.

These, then, are the themes of this book. Our starting point is actually near the bottom of the diagram, which is where we find the more usual focus of food and nutritional science. The traditional emphasis continues in much teaching and research, that is to say on the properties and uses of foods rather than on the nutritional problems of populations. Part of the purpose of this book is to present a reverse perspective – to put the problems of people first and see what questions they prompt about nutrition. To reverse the traditional perspective of nutrition in this way is not, of course, to say that everything done previously was mistaken. What we would argue, though, is that if one constantly approaches a subject from the same point of view, important insights may be missed, and received views may not be adequately questioned. For example, to tackle the question of how much food human beings require we first ask what kind of life those individuals lead, and what physiological functions, therefore, does their food intake have to support?

If the science of nutrition has any central concept, it is surely this notion of nutrient requirements. The initial impetus for the subject came from nineteenth-century attempts to define those requirements, and in many quarters, that approach is still important. The process of revising estimates of energy and protein requirements continues unabated, and the problem of fixing them remains apparently unresolved. What has changed since the early days is that originally pronouncements about nutrient requirements were made by individual scientists and were based on their own research; now, similar pronouncements emanate from committees of experts convened by governments or international agencies and to a large extent reflect the experts' selection of scientific evidence and of theory (Rivers and Payne, 1982).

Despite the authority and influence associated with some of these figures, the concept of a 'nutrient requirement' remains somewhat intangible. Discrepancies between estimates, and the revisions that are made from time to time, do not seem to reflect differences in technique or theory, but may have more to do with political pressures or changing social valuations of the acceptability of particular intake levels. For example, successive estimates of food energy requirements made by the US National Academy of Sciences for a moderately active man with a body weight of 70kg have been as follows (NAS 1943, 1958, etc.):

> 12.5 MJ (3000 kcal) in 1943;
> 13.4 MJ (3200 kcal) in 1958;
> 11.7 MJ (2800 kcal) in 1968;
> 11.3 MJ (2700 kcal) in 1974.

The 16 per cent fall in estimated requirements since 1958 is not the result of improvements in the process of estimation, nor of any factor such as change in levels of activity, but must be attributed more vaguely to climates of opinion and perhaps concern about obesity.

Nonetheless, the questions 'how much food does a man/woman/child need?' and 'what are the reasons for and consequences of failing to meet that need?' remain central to agricultural development. We set out below some of the issues involved in answering them and the problems raised thereby. We use a series of short case studies (from different parts of the world) to illustrate them.

Food energy and agrarian ecology

Lack of progress in attempts to define human energy and nutrient needs illustrates one reason why it is useful to think in terms of the level of nutrition needed to maintain the functional capacity of the body. If we take the traditional view of a nutrient requirement as the minimal amount of nutrient needed to maintain a given physiological state such as 'health', then we are faced with the problem of specifying that state. And although health and well-being are certainly to be valued as social goals, the utility of health as a reference criterion is limited by our inability to define a state of ideal health which an adequate nutrient intake should sustain.

The social nature of the definition of health has been

frequently discussed elsewhere (Illich, 1976; McKeown, 1979), its use as a criterion for fixing energy requirement is particularly complicated by the fact that it seems impossible to identify a healthy population. As one official body states, most of their recommendations on food energy are based on measurements of what actual populations eat, assuming that these populations are healthy. However, they point out that: 'Many groups of people ... living in the industrialized countries are obese. On the other hand some groups living in developing countries are small in stature, light and thin, yet may not be physically less healthy because of their different body size' (FAO/WHO, 1973).

Another approach is to attempt the definition of energy requirement in terms of the maintenance of a specified physiological state, disregarding notions such as 'health' and this leads to the apparently more precise concept of 'nutrient balance', a deceptively simple notion which has been widely applied in animal nutrition (Blaxter, 1967).

Obviously, in the non-pregnant adult animal, nutrient intake and expenditure must match if the body content of the nutrient is not to rise or be depleted. The problem is that balance can be achieved over a range of intakes through adaptations of various kinds. Thus the question 'which level of nutrient balance is preferred?' is inescapable, and can only be answered by referring back to 'health'.

The balance method is thus no more objective than the health criterion. The decision about what level of equilibrium or for children, what rate of growth, and hence what degree of positive balance, will be regarded as a norm remains entirely subjective unless we are prepared to specify a particular set of desired functions and a set of undesirable symptoms we wish to avoid. The decision which is usually made (albeit not always explicitly) is to say that we prefer the levels and growth rates which are typical of western developed countries, though we are discovering that these are not without disadvantage for health.

It is in order to avoid such ambiguities and difficulties that this book uses 'functional' criteria of the adequacy of food intakes. From this point of view, malnutrition is defined as a state in which the physical function of an individual is impaired to the

Table 1.1 *Energy intakes of New Guinea adults*

Village		Body weight	Energy intake per day	
		kg	*MJ*	*kcal*
Kaul (coastal location)	males	56	8.12	1940
	females	47	5.94	1420
Lafa (highland location)	males	57	10.54	2520
	females	51	8.79	2100

Source: Norgan *et al*. 1974.

point where she or he can no longer maintain adequate perform-ance in such processes as growth, pregnancy, lactation, physical work, or resisting and recovering from disease. The notion of an adequate level of performance is itself not a simple one. However, it avoids the rather greater difficulties of talking about adequate levels of health if, in the first instance, we use it to mean the achievement of a sustainable mode of existence. Thus, for example, to avoid malnutrition, members of a farming family must be able to do physical work on their land and crops, sufficient not only to secure their immediate food needs, but to sustain productivity over long periods, and to survive through bad years as well as good. They must in addition be able to adjust total production from their resources to keep pace with the demographic changes (numbers of dependants and number of productive adults) in the family itself.

In taking this approach, we regard dietary energy as the most likely limiting factor. This does not imply that vitamin and other deficiencies do not occur, or are of minor consequence. Rather we are suggesting that the avoidance of energy constraints is a necessary even if not always a sufficient condition for avoiding malnutrition.

In the context of agriculture, the problem of energy deficiency is quite a subtle one, partly because of the wide range of different farming ecologies that can be successfully exploited, and partly because we have to look at equilibrium situations where the working capacity of adult family members is both the outcome of a particular level of food consumption, and the labour input to the production system which generates the food. Viable equilibrium can therefore be maintained over a range of levels of intake and output. As an example, Table 1.1 shows the average food energy consumption levels of men and women in two villages in New Guinea.

The people of both villages had similar and generally good states of health, without any signs of malnutrition. However, members of the coastal community needed to devote only small amounts of labour to their gardens, and despite a plentiful source of fish, rarely bothered to go and catch them. Most of their day was spent in leisure and socialising. The highland community, by contrast, lived and worked on steep mountain slopes, and spent several hours a day in fairly heavy labour. The two situations are both successful from the point of view of health and survival. Food energy needs are different, however, and if malnutrition did occur at some future time because of limited land access, or because of some climatic event, it would do so at different levels of food consumption.

Consider now rice cultivation. It is estimated that dryland rice requires approximately 130 man-days of labour input per hectare in one environment (Bayliss Smith 1981), corresponding to a work input of about 390 MJ per hectare. It will yield on average about 15,000 MJ net edible yield of rice – about 1000 kg – so the ratio of energy output to input is 38:1. This is not an unusual figure, since according to Leach (1975) energy ratios for pre-industrial crops are generally in the range from 13 to 38. When food energy production in a pre-industrial society is at or below the lower end of that range, it is likely that not enough food is being produced to support non-agricultural work such as water-carrying or house-building, and to support non-working members (old people and children), so malnutrition in the sense of functional failure becomes increasingly probable.

Changes in energy needs over time

At this level of analysis, the picture presented is of a simple, static equilibrium, with energy flows averaged over time, and no account taken of the effects of either regular seasonal factors, or irregular unpredictable hazards. Seasonal factors may impose two kinds of restriction, in the first place related to *time* intensity. Certain tasks must be carried out in specific seasonal time periods and this may impose a lower limit on the number of working adults or their equivalents per hectare necessary to secure a given type of crop. Secondly, *work* intensity may impose limitations bearing in mind that the physical work required for certain tasks may be much greater than average and may only be sustainable by individuals with a high level of physical fitness, i.e. good nutritional status, and freedom from disease or injury.

Further, agricultural seasons are not always the same; there are good years and bad years. Survival in bad years means either the ability to achieve a surplus during good years, with some means to carry this over as stored food, as cash, or as assets which may be collateral on loans, or some other opportunities for converting labour resources to food or cash by alternative employment.

An additional, longer-term result of the passage of time is that the size and demographic structure of the family will change: total food needs increase steadily as successive children are born, but later the children grow up and contribute to the family's labour power. Together, then, the influence of seasonal cycles and family development is such that we need a dynamic view of the whole food system, of the functions which take place within it, and of the environmental and temporal changes which form its context.

A village in Burkina Faso, West Africa, where millet is the principal crop, illustrates one kind of sharply seasonal contrast. In this area, the dry season is a long one; it is followed by a relatively short period when the soils are sufficiently softened by the rain to be workable, and when crops must be sown. During this period, therefore, long hours of labour are necessary. The time intensity and work intensity of the effort people must make are both high. Human energy expenditures are, as a result, comparable to those found only in coal mining in more industrialised economies. By contrast, during the dry season there is little work to be done and

Table 1.2   *Energy expenditures of farmers in an Upper Volta village*

		Energy expended per day	
		MJ	kcal
Dry season	{ women	9.7	2320
	men	10.1	2410
Wet season	{ women	12.1	2890
	men	14.4	3460

Sources: Bleiberg *et al.* (1980); Brun *et al.* 1981.

energy expenditures are low. The men in particular have a very sedentary lifestyle and their energy expenditure drops sharply (Table 1.2).

This example shows that when we look at energy expenditure and food supply on a single occasion, or indeed, averaged out over a year, we can tell very little about the adequacy of diet, or the likelihood of malnutrition. For these West African villagers, malnutrition might consist of inability to meet peak labour demands because of either insufficient food available to balance expenditure *at that time*, or because of body stores insufficiently replenished since the previous working season.

In all probability, people using this kind of production system face problems of both time and work intensity, and their responses are partly behavioural and social, partly physiological: the periods of peak work output, which may be quite short in time, are sustained partly at the expense of body energy stores. Thus people lose weight, and then regain it during a subsequent period when work output is dramatically reduced, but food intake is maintained at the previous level, or even increased. Figure 1.2 shows these effects as they have been observed in Gambia. This country is also in West Africa, and the seasonal ecology is similar (though less extreme) to that of Burkina Faso (Fox 1953). Periods of peak energy expenditure are associated with harvesting, and with soil preparation and planting.

Obviously, there are physiological limits to the extent of this cyclic process: if too much weight is lost, perhaps because of a

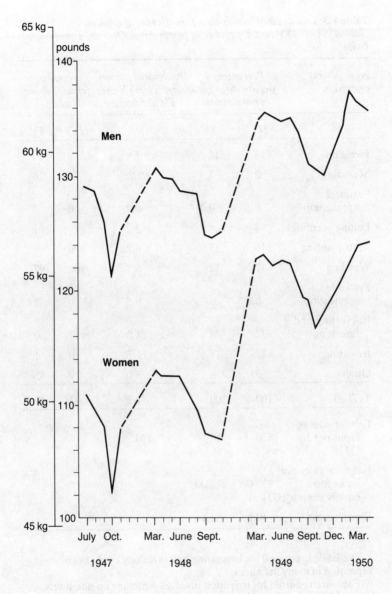

Figure 1.2 Fluctuations in adult body weight by season in a Gambian village

Source: Fox 1953

Table 1.3   *Analysis of labour time for different operations of cultivation of HYV and TV paddy in North Arcot District, Tamil Nadu, India*

Agricultural operation	Percentage of person-days spent in the operation		Additional person-days for HYV over TV per hectare	Percentage of female labour used	
	HYV	TV		HYV	TV
Ploughing	18	18	5.9	0	0
Manuring	2	3	1.2	22	26
Fertiliser application	0.5	0.4	0.2	0	3
Pulling seedlings	4	4	2.2	17	21
Transplanting	15	15	6.2	100	98
Weeding	12	12	3.7	100	97
Pesticide application	0.2	0.1	0.5	0	2
Harvesting and threshing[1]	32	28	24.8	57	60
Irrigation[2]	13	15	1.5	0	1
Others	3	4	3.0	29	55
TOTAL	100	100	41.2	47	47
Labour energy input per ha (MJ)[3]	830	710	120		
Net edible rice per ha as food energy output (GJ)	33,000	24,000			
Energy ratio	40:1	34:1			

Notes:
[1] The labour required for harvesting and threshing could not be separated in many instances.
[2] The work required for irrigation involves switching on pump sets, waiting for electricity, or operating the kavalai.
[3] Labour input is estimated roughly as 3MJ per person-day.

Source: Based on Table 14.2 in Chinnappa and Silva 1977.

poor previous season, then peak work output may be impaired, reducing the potential for next year's crop still further. Despite recent research into the nutrition and physiological work, most experimental measurements have sought to measure the steady-state behaviour of individuals and animals. Thus relatively little is known about responses to fluctuations in intake or work output, or about the body's energy and nutrient storage mechanisms. Yet the latter may have a very much larger role than previously realised for key vitamins and minerals as well as for energy (Longhurst and Payne, 1979). Lacking knowledge of these, we cannot assess the risks of malnutrition for people living in highly seasonal environments.

Data on seasonal energy relationships in the context of rice cropping is available from the North Arcot district of Tamil Nadu state (India). Table 1.3 shows a breakdown of the time spent on various stages in the agricultural cycle, both for traditional (TV) and high yielding (HYV) varieties of rice (Chinnappa and Silva, 1977). The change to HYVs in this region increased yields to the point where a family of five people could theoretically meet its basic energy needs by cultivating only 0.5 ha. This estimate is based on a food energy output of 33,000 MJ per hectare annually. The ratio of energy output to input was then 40:1, which is slightly higher than before HYV rice was introduced.

It is clear, then, that a family which adopted HYVs did not require any additional labour to meet its own food requirements. But since yields were greater, these requirements could be met from less land. The remainder of the land formerly used could then produce a surplus for sale, but only if more labour was employed. In practice, most families adopting HYVs were those with the larger holdings, and they secured the extra labour by hiring workers from among the smaller cultivators and landless families. That particularly affected the employment of women for tasks occupying short, intensive seasons such as transplanting, weeding and harvesting (Table 1.3), which is significant in relation to a seasonal peak occurring locally in the birth rate (Chambers *et al.*, 1981). At the time when they need to be working in the fields, many mothers have very young infants whom they should be breast-feeding. This can mean that feeds are hurried, or badly spaced, and babies do not get enough (Devkota, 1981; Rickleton, 1981).

Not only do work patterns and birth rates commonly vary markedly with season, but so do infectious diseases. When seasonal peaks of infection coincide with times of food shortage and hard work, the consequences of malnutrition may be compounded. The greatest regular seasonal impact on rural society is often due to infections and parasites (Bradley, 1981), and these have strong interactions with nutrition.

Clearly, disease can be both a cause and a result of poverty. It affects the efficiency of work, and that is one of several reasons why the previous discussion of the minimum energy inputs needed to feed a family from a rice crop is a considerable simplification. In practice, the family's survival would depend on exceeding these levels, so that there is a margin to allow for times when individuals are not working because of illness, as well as to allow for grain lost in store (5–10 per cent) or retained for seed. Furthermore, although the rice could supply all the energy and protein needs of the family, it would not fully supply vitamin and mineral needs. The family would thus have to invest more labour either in farm production of vegetables and other foods, or in paid employment, or in an increased production of rice for sale and exchange.

Very often, the levels of labour input referred to earlier would need to be increased by up to 50 per cent to cover the needs for exchange purposes, and to provide an insurance against poor harvests and crop levels. This insurance investment would depend upon the level of ecological variability of the region. In an extremely variable climate such as that of Burkina Faso, the traditional practice before 1920 was to aim for a level of stocks after harvest equivalent to 2–3 years' grain consumption (George, 1980). However, the ability to make any insurance clearly depends on the labour and land resources available. In South Asia the marginal farm family with land restricted to less than their subsistence production needs will be in a precarious situation with regard to bad years and the landless even more so.

Family development

Seasonal changes in food supply must be studied in relation to the longer-term cycle of the family's demographic expansion, as children are born and grow up. During the first year or two of marriage, both parents are usually able to contribute in labour or other economic activity, particularly if the timing of pregnancy is such that the women can still work during the time-intensive part of the production cycle. Earning or production capacity will then be high in relation to the number of family members to be supported, and the economic dependency ratio is low.

Things may become more difficult as the number of children increases and if and when they are at school. Later, as the children take on more and more work, the economic burden carried by each working members of the family eases. Food energy needs in a family and the number of workers necessary to support that family are thus constantly changing over time.

Young children require relatively large amounts of dietary energy. A one-year-old child is one-fifth the weight of an adult, but his/her energy intake will be about half the adult level. Somehow the young child has to take in a relatively large amount of food. Much depends on the frequency with which a child is fed and on the amounts of milk she/he is given. Rutishauser (1974), working in Uganda, found that the factors associated with a good energy intake in children under two years old were:

1. breast-feeding continued while other foods were introduced
2. three or more non-breast feeds per day
3. 'good appetite', i.e. absence of infection.

It is of critical importance that the mother or whoever cares for a child should have sufficient time in the working day to help that child to feed, and in some cases, to prepare special items for him/her, because even though the family diet may have a good nutrient density, certain nutrient-rich items may be too spicy or hard to handle. The high growth rates and high relative energy needs of young children require frequent concentrated feeds, yet the lifestyle of many poor families makes this extremely difficult to achieve, especially at seasons when work is highly time-intensive (Wheeler, 1982).

We have already noted that adult agricultural workers sometimes lose weight during peak labour seasons and then regain it at times of year when there is more food available and less work. This fluctuation may be regarded as a satisfactory adaptation to a changing environment. However, if pregnant and lactating women suffer energy deficits during periods of hard physical work, their offspring will be smaller and more vulnerable (Paul *et al.*, 1979). Evidence that Asian women's energy status does fluctuate seasonally is provided by the observations of Chowdhury *et al.* (1981) in Bangladesh. There, the women of landless families tend to lose weight during the August–October period, when the highest labour demands for rice cultivation are just over, and the price of rice is highest. Should these women be pregnant or lactating at that season, the risk of malnutrition to both mother and child is increased.

Illness may temporarily alter nutrient requirements. Gastrointestinal diseases often lead to malabsorption of food, and many illnesses lead to tissue breakdown or blood loss to a varying degree. During the acute phase of an illness, nutrient utilisation

Table 1.4 *Food energy needs and labour available at three stages in the development of a family*

	Food energy needs MJ/year	Adult male labour equivalent	Ratio of energy need to labour available
Woman and man, 1 child under 2 years	9,500	1.8	5.3
Woman and man, 1 child under 2, 1 child between 2 & 3, 1 child between 4 & 5	14,500	1.8	8.0
Woman and man, 1 child under 5, 1 child between 8 & 10*, 1 child between 10 & 12*, 1 child between 12 & 15**	21,500	3.6	6.0

Notes: * assumed equivalent to 0.5 of an economically active man;
 ** assumed equivalent to 0.8 of an economically active man.

Food systems and needs 35

falls so there is need for some increment during recovery. Clearly, this is a more serious matter for children than for adults; they need nutrients and energy for growth, and also their body nutrient reserves are small. This may be seen particularly in children with acute fevers or gastro-enteritis, who can become wasted and also dehydrated very fast, unless there is a determined effort to keep their fluid and food intake as high as possible (Mata, 1977; Briscoe, 1979).

For a great variety of reasons, then, human nutritional needs vary markedly throughout life. There is a steady fall in necessary intake in proportion to body weight until adulthood, after which the appropriate level of intake depends greatly on work and activity, and on physiological stresses, of which the most important for women is pregnancy.

Human requirements for food are not constant, but vary with the development of family groups as much as for individuals. Table 1.4 presents typical figures for a particular family at three stages in its development, and shows how there may be a critical period when the children are all young. At this stage, energy needs in relation to the labour available to meet them peak sharply. During this period, there is a maximum likelihood of malnutrition occurring, particularly at the most intensive stages of the seasonal cycle. Thus the focus of many nutrition programmes on the problems of young children makes sense not only because of the vulnerability of the children themselves, but also because of the vulnerability of the family group as a whole while the children are young.

To understand the prospects of the family group in more detail, however, we need to look beyond the children and enquire whether the family owns and cultivates its own land, and whether it is able to hire farm workers at especially busy times of year, since that is an important way of dealing with peak energy demands. Families with little or no land of their own will often be in more critical situations. Most difficult of all are the seasonal problems of families with small plots of their own, but who are also partly dependent on paid work. For them, the best opportunities for farm employment are likely to coincide with the heaviest demands of their own crops.

Any investigation of the problems faced by such people should also take account of agricultural developments which may modify the magnitude and timing of seasonal effects, crop varieties and irrigation.

All our examples so far have been of rural agricultural households, but the principles could be applied to other groups such as urban unskilled labouring families, plantation workers, pastoralists, fishing families, and so on. Investigation of social or economic differences, of the effects of technical change, or seasonal constraints, and the problems of family development, entails classifying families by land ownership and tenure, by dependence on markets, and by major sources of income. This would be an example of what is referred to later (Chapter 6) as a 'functional classification' of the population being studied. Examining the prevalence rates for malnutrition season by season for each of the groups identified, enables us to study malnutrition on a comparative basis. Because of the importance of this approach, we shall repeatedly return to such questions as land tenure and cropping patterns. First, though, it is necessary to consider certain other nutritional concepts, and these are the subject for the next two chapters.

2 Defining malnutrition*

Comparative views

Malnutrition, according to the previous chapter, should be understood in terms of failures of bodily functions. The conditions under which it occurs must be appreciated as specific to particular localities, with characteristic agricultural ecologies and work patterns. People adapt to a great variety of dietary and work regimes, and this sometimes involves modifications in body size, levels of physical activity, and metabolic changes. Detecting malnutrition is a matter of detecting degrees of such change which carry unacceptable penalties in terms of hunger, illness, dysfunction and risk of dysfunction. We shall return later to the implications of the word 'unacceptable', and merely note that these ideas may together be characterised as an 'individual adaptability view' of malnutrition.

It is this view upon which the present book is based, and to avoid misunderstanding, we need to compare it with other concepts, of which the most important is the 'fixed genetic potential view'. The basic premise here is that there is an optimal or preferred state of health, fixed for each individual, and determined by his or her genetic potential for growth, resistance to disease, longevity, and so on. It is assumed that everyone

---

*This chapter is based on material prepared by Elizabeth Dowler and Philip Payne. See Dowler *et al.*, 1982.

could and should achieve their full genetic potential and that malnutrition starts as soon as there is any departure from the preferred state. We cannot measure human genetic potential, however, so it is further assumed that the standards of body size and food intake observed in 'well-fed' and 'healthy' populations approximate to this optimum.

It may be useful to compare these contrasting views with one which gained acceptance two decades ago. Jelliffe (1966, p.8) regarded malnutrition as, 'a pathological state resulting from a relative or absolute deficiency or excess of one or more essential nutrients, this state being clinically manifested or detected only by biochemical, anthropometric or physiological tests'.

Two points made by this definition should be especially noted. Firstly, it implies that deficiency or excess of nutrients is the major cause of the pathological state referred to, whereas we would now wish to emphasise the role of many other contributory causes (Chapter 4). Secondly, Jelliffe states that malnutrition can be detected *only* by biochemical, anthropometric or physiological tests. It cannot be deduced from an individual's level of food intake, nor can it be estimated from the average intake of a population.

In this second respect, the individual adaptability view and Jelliffe's definition are in close agreement, and stand in opposition to the assumption often made that malnutrition can be inferred whenever intakes of nutrients fall below certain fixed levels. Many statistics which purport to represent the number of malnourished people in the world (or in specific countries) actually represent the number with low food intakes. We cited one example in the previous chapter of two societies of apparently healthy populations whose energy intakes were markedly different. We also mentioned the importance of food in cultural and social exchange, and suggested that an individual's ability to obtain food may be a good indication of his integration with society. Thus the number of people whose food intakes fall below a certain level may be an important statistic for measuring poverty or social differentiation (Chapter 6); it may often include some malnourished people and some who are seasonally hungry. But whatever its social significance, such a figure does not measure the prevalence of malnutrition in its scientific sense.

The manifestations of malnutrition vary. In what follows, unless otherwise stated, we are referring to protein-energy malnutrition.

In a population with relatively low food intakes, only a minority of children may show clinical symptoms of malnutrition such as oedema, fatty liver, hair and skin changes, or severe muscle wasting, but others may very well be affected especially with regard to their vulnerability to infection. Other clinical signs include diminished subcutaneous fat, and low body weight relative to height. Beaton and Bengoa (1976) and Alleyne *et al.* (1977) give useful descriptions of these signs and symptoms, and of the recommended methods for weighing children and taking measurements of height (or length of infants), and of arm circumference.

But the question then arises: by what standard should we decide whether body weights are low? If this is one of the populations cited in the previous chapter where it is 'normal' for people to lose weight markedly during certain seasons, are we in a position to make allowance for that? If the average height of the people is unusually small, do we interpret this as an abnormality and call it 'stunting', or might it be an 'adaptation' to environmental conditions? If the people are New Guinea tribesmen whose children are relatively free from illness but whose environment has unusual features, 'adaptation' would seem the appropriate description. But with Indian village children whose growth is checked by episodes of serious illness from which recovery is slowed by low food intake, 'undernutrition' would seem a more relevant description. Between these two extremes there are many uncertain categories. Moreover, we still do not know very much about how to distinguish populations going through 'normal' seasonal cycles of weight loss and recovery from those whose body reserves had been diminished by a downward spiral of impoverishment. Thus questions about how we interpret small body size or low body weight are particularly important.

What we really need to know about are the relationships between body size and such functions as immune competence, mental function, physical work capacity, or the likelihood of survival. All these functions are interrelated, but the links between them are not well understood. As Chapter 4 will demonstrate, little is known about the relationship of anthropometric data to mortality risk and morbidity, but this suggests that we shall probably never be able to locate fixed points on, say, a weight-for-age scale which will sharply divide individuals at risk from those we regard as normal. To the extent that such cut-off points can be established at all, they will probably only be valid for specified population groups living in particular localities. So, for example, it seems impossible to classify mortality risks for a group of children in Zaire using anthropometric criteria which worked well for children in Bangladesh (Kasango Project Team 1983).

Screening and anthropometry

The practical importance of establishing and defining criteria for labelling people as 'malnourished' can be illustrated by discussing the problems of selecting a subgroup of the 'malnourished' for treatment or intervention.

Despite the difficulties of classification, in any practical situation where action is contemplated, there will be a need to have some procedure for comparing risks and for allocating resources. We might in some circumstances consider that risk of death is the most important criterion and confine ourselves to this. We shall find, however, that even in such a relatively simple situation, classifying individuals as 'at risk' will depend not only on the risk relationship but also on the resources available and the logistics involved.

For example, Chen *et al.* (1980) have reported the experience of a sample of 2019 children in Bangladesh. Their weights, heights and arm circumference measurements were recorded when they were one year old. After two years, during which only treatment for diarrhoea was available, 112 of them had died.

We can employ the data about these children to show what the effect would be using two different variables, weight-for-age and weight-for-height, as a basis for allocating some more effective treatment. To do this, we imagine two kinds of situation, in both of which it has been decided to use anthropometry for screening the group – that is, as a means of selecting individuals who will be given food rations or provided with some kind of treatment aimed at rehabilitation. We shall assume that resources are limited, and that the treatment, if given, is equally effective in reducing the risk to a level close to the minimum, however severely the recipient is affected. The two situations are:

1. The population to be screened is of fixed and known size, such as an entire refugee camp; our problem is simply to decide who gets treated and who does not.
2. The 2019 children are just a sample of a very much larger group, and there is a continuous queue of applicants for screening.

Table 2.1 shows the numbers of children in various categories

Table 2.1 *Numbers of children out of a population of 2019, who would have been identified and treated for malnutrition, using two different indicators[1]*

	Number identified as in need of treatment	Number of preventable deaths[2]	Number of false positives treated[3]	Deaths pre-vented per treatment
Weight-for-age				
<60% of reference	427	48	379	0.112
<75% of reference	1473	92	1381	0.062
Weight-for-height				
<70% of reference	75	11	64	0.147
<80% of reference	641	39	602	0.061
<90% of reference	1620	92	1528	0.057
Treatment of the total population	2019	112	1907	0.055

Notes:
[1] Data taken from Tables 1 and 2 in Chen *et al*. 1980, which consists of a study of mortality rates in 2019 Bangladeshi children during a two-year period following a survey of nutritional status.
[2] This is the number of children who actually died in the group studied by Chen *et al*.
[3] Number of children who survived.

of weight-for-age and weight-for-height whose deaths in our theoretical case would be prevented if they were selected for treatment. It will be noticed that instead of quoting the actual weights of the children, we quote them as percentages of a reference weight or standard – in this case the 'Harvard' standard. This represents the average weight of a large sample of apparently healthy children at the same age as the individuals being measured. Recording data as 'percentage of reference' for each individual's age allows older and younger groups to be compared directly, or allows the data for all the children to be amalgamated. (We consider this practice in more detail in Chapter 4.)

In this example, those children who are below a stated percentage level are selected for treatment and the second column in the table shows how many would be involved. Thus if 60 per cent of reference weight-for-age were taken as the critical point and if all children under that were treated, this would entail a total of 427 treatments. Of these, 48 would be given to children otherwise likely to die, so there would be a ratio of one 'genuine' to 8.9 'false' positives being treated.* Obviously, if the critical point on the reference scale were raised from 60 towards 100 per cent, the numbers of treatments that would have to be given out would rise and eventually cover the whole population. The ratio of 'false' to 'genuine' subjects treated would also increase. Supposing the group of 2019 children comprised a complete community and the critical level depended on the number of treatments available. If there were resources for, say, 500 treatments, a point slightly above 60 per cent would give the best allocation, reaching over 50 children who would otherwise die; 1000 treatments would reach 80, and so on.

If weight-for-height were to be used, the situation would be somewhat different. At low critical points, such as 70 per cent reference weight-for-height, the selection is much more specific than by using weight-for-age. It excludes many false positives,

---

*The notion of a false positive here refers to mortality and not to mortality plus morbidity, where the concept might have to be modified.

and gives lower ratios of 'false' to 'genuine' subjects treated; however this specificity is at the expense of also excluding many 'genuine' subjects as well – only 11 deaths would be prevented.

If we again consider what happens when 500 treatments are available, we find that they would have to be allocated on the basis of about 75 per cent of reference weight-for-height, but that only 30 of them would then go to children who would otherwise die. With 1000 treatments, we would need a cut-off point at rather less than 85 per cent, and 60 lives would be saved, and so on. This, of course, assumes that the kind of risk assessed by these two variables, weight-for-age and weight-for-height is the same: that high risk cases identified by both would respond equally well to the same treatment.

The other situation, where we envisage a continuous queue of children being brought for treatment, is more complex. If the rate at which individuals can be treated (the rate of admission for rehabilitation, or the rate at which food supplements can be delivered) is fixed, we might want the critical point for screening and selection to be that which identified individuals for treatment at a matching rate. On the other hand, we would want as low a ratio of treatments to preventable deaths as possible. The second requirement would be satisfied by using 70 per cent of reference weight-for-height as the cut-off point. But then the first requirement might only be realised if the measurement were carried out faster, for example by employing more people to do it, thereby selecting more children for treatment per unit of time.

We have elaborated this example to illustrate that however artificially we constrain the system, we cannot expect to find a unique answer to the question of how to classify the malnourished. It would of course be convenient if a particular percentage of reference weight-for-age could be taken as an unambiguous cut-off point or boundary between 'severe' and 'moderate' malnutrition, or between 'malnutrition' and 'normality'. Some systems for classifying anthropometric data imply distinctions of this sort, but the example shows that wherever we draw a dividing line, some individuals who are not at risk will be selected for treatment while others who are at risk will not. Thus in practice, the precise percentage of reference weight we take as a dividing line or cut-off point is chosen according to our resources, circumstances and purpose.

It is clear how the resources available, and how the circumstances of a refugee camp or, alternatively, an endless queue of children, may alter procedures. As to purpose, we may compare this example of screening to select children for treatment, with several other purposes for which body weights and heights may be recorded.

For example, when the illness of a single child is being diagnosed, his weight might well be noted, but it is clear from the figures in Table 2.1 that weight-for-age would not signify much by itself. If the child has been attending a clinic regularly, and his weight has been plotted on a growth chart each time, any faltering of growth will be readily recognised. But the clinic staff will also examine the child, looking for evidence of infection as well as for classical signs of malnutrition such as oedema (though these signs are present only in severe cases). Enquiries might also be made about the child's home circumstances, to assess whether food has been in short supply, whether there are particular hygiene problems, or whether the mother is well enough, or has sufficient time, to prepare food for the child. In other words, to form a clear view of an individual's condition, one requires a combination of different kinds of evidence, and as always, diagnosis of an *individual* condition and needs is by a combination of clinical experience and measurement.

By contrast, where there are large numbers of people to cope with, screening procedures such as we have envisaged being used in a refugee camp must usually be employed. Then, individuals have to be selected for treatment on the basis of only one or two routinely applied tests. In these circumstances, we know that many of those selected will not need treatment, and some urgent cases will be missed. Thus the problem is to design the test so that it selects as well as possible within its limitations.

Yet another purpose which is sometimes served by recording children's body weights and heights is monitoring and surveillance. The aim here is to identify social groups at nutritional risk, or to check whether there is a trend for nutritional status in a population to improve or worsen over time. In surveys of this kind, we again look at the number of individuals whose weights or heights fall below a stated percentage of some reference level. However, we are not now worried by 'false positives' included in the numbers we count, provided that nutritional position of the two is clearly and fairly shown. Thus we may decide to record the proportion of children who are below, say, 85 per cent reference weight-for-age, comparing farmers' children with children in the families of labourers, plantation workers, artisans, and so on. The choice of the 85 per cent reference level would not necessarily reflect any nutritional benchmark, nor would it be determined by the resources available to support some kind of action. It would be chosen because in some social groups, many children are below this level, while in others, most children are above it. If we counted the number of children whose weight relative to age was below 110 per cent of reference, contrasts would disappear because nearly everybody would be in this category.

These examples of different ways in which anthropometric data could be interpreted and used reflect the assumption associated with the 'adaptability view' that an individual's nutritional condition cannot be directly measured. Data on weight, height, arm circumference and so on are therefore indirect or proxy descriptions whose relationship with 'risk of dysfunction' is a complex one. In particular, measurements above which risk is uniformly low, but below which the adaptive capacity of the body has been exceeded.

The 'genetic potential view', by contrast, stresses maximisation of potential for growth, which means that measurements of height and weight are identified much more closely with the individual's nutritional condition. So after allowing for the proportion of the population whose small body sizes are genetically determined, any deficiency in height and weight is regarded as evidence of malnutrition. This leads to more people being counted as malnourished than under most of the other procedures discussed in this chapter.

Some policy implications

These differences in the definition and classification of malnutrition are carried over, not surprisingly, into policy recommendations. One approach, appropriate to the conditions in many low-income countries where death rates are high and resources are scarce, is to concentrate on those conditions in which lives are threatened most immediately and directly.

A much more comprehensive approach is sometimes encountered, however, especially among those who take the 'genetic potential' view. One early exponent was John Boyd-Orr, whose concept of adequate nutrition was 'a state of well-being such that no improvement can be effected by a change in diet' (Boyd-Orr, 1936, p.12). Interpreting 'well-being' in terms of a fairly ample and varied food intake, Boyd-Orr made surveys of how much food people in Britain could afford to buy during the economic depression of the early 1930s and estimated that about half the population was below this adequate intake – more than 20 million people (Boyd-Orr, 1936, p.49). When he became the first Director-General of FAO, Boyd-Orr initiated its first World Food Survey, which found that over 50 per cent of the world's population lived in 'calorie-deficient countries' (FAO, 1946). This was regularly interpreted as meaning that half, and by 1950, two-thirds of mankind were malnourished (Poleman, 1981).

A recent instance of estimates derived from the view that every individual should achieve his or her full genetic potential for growth was a statement attributed to Dr C. Gopalan which attracted attention in the western press (*Guardian*, 1982; *Economist*, 1983). Of the 23 million babies born in India each year, he said, 4 million die in childhood and 16 million experience malnutrition to a greater or lesser extent, leaving only 3 million to grow completely unscathed into healthy adults.

These viewpoints have validity as general social commentaries about the persistence of levels of nutrition which ought to be regarded as unacceptable. But there are dangers in using such all-embracing views of malnutrition and the high estimates of the numbers of malnourished people to which they lead as a sufficient basis for identifying policy. The kinds of policies proposed are likely to be general and non-discriminatory in character and their effectiveness will be judged on the basis of their impact on the *average* levels of nutrition of the population. The total benefit may be large, but it will be widely spread, so that even those whose needs are slight will experience some. In addition, of course greatly increased total food production is usually seen as a precondition. The difficulty with this kind of policy, however, is that most benefit is usually felt in the 'middle ranks' of society, and the bottom 5 or 10 per cent may be little affected, and are unlikely to recover the priority that their greater degree of nutritional deprivation should entitle them to. In addition, there is a very real likelihood that the problem of malnutrition comes to be seen as so large and so demanding of resources for increased consumption and welfare as to be impossible of solution within any reasonable time frame without sacrificing other development objectives. To plan welfare measures effectively requires either a more discriminating view of which groups within the population are most in need or the acceptance of the very high costs of interventions which do not discriminate.

A different policy approach is suggested by saying that instead of seeking 'the greatest happiness for the greatest number', one should demand, more modestly, 'the least amount of avoidable suffering for all'. Still other policies would result from suggesting that where some suffering cannot be avoided, as with hunger in times of food shortage, that suffering should be distributed 'as equally as possible'. Karl Popper (1945), whose point this is, goes on to argue that it aids clarity 'if we formulate our demands negatively, i.e. if we demand the elimination of suffering rather than the promotion of happiness' – or health.

The change in emphasis in political action which the minimisation of and equalisation of unavoidable suffering would imply is important. This is because the nature and intensity of nutritional deprivation is highly differentiated as between different groups of people and between various causes of dietary inadequacy. Action either to minimise or to equalise suffering might therefore start by identifying the worst cases. This might then lead to the implementation of measures that are specifically designed to change their circumstances. The point can be illustrated in

Table 2.2   *Malnutrition in children aged under 5 measured in Rwanda and Kenya*

	Severe malnutrition (below 60% of reference weight-for-age, or 70% weight-for-height)	Moderate malnutrition (between 60% and 75% reference weight-for-age, or between 70% and 80% weight-for-height)
Rwanda, % of children under 5	9.8	44.9
Kenya, % of children under 5	1.0	25.0

Source: FAO 1977.

principle, though not in historical fact, by data from anthropometric surveys quoted by FAO (1977), and particularly by figures from two African countries (Table 2.2).

In Rwanda, it would clearly be important to plan policy interventions around the 10 per cent of children who are severely malnourished. In Kenya, policy could be based on a broader definition of malnutrition – we could take 75 per cent weight-for-age as a cut-off point without having a problem which is unmanageable in a given political economy – but we would still need to investigate the 1 per cent of severely malnourished children to check whether they represent concentrations of poverty for which resources for special measures might be needed.

As conditions in a country improve, and if pockets of severe deprivation can be eliminated, cut-off points for defining malnutrition can also be raised. In Britain in the 1930s, Boyd-Orr was right to use a high standard because many people in the nation were already well nourished, and as he pointed out, resources were available which could raise everybody to that level. But to apply the same standards in modern India is to present planners with a task too large for the resources at their disposal; more seriously, it hides the nutritionally urgent problems in the immensity of the less nutritionally urgent.

Scientific models

In discussing the interpretation of anthropometric data, Trow-bridge (1979) recalls the story of the blind men who encounter an elephant and have to identify it from the shapes they can feel. Each man touches a different part of the elephant and comes to a different conclusion about the nature of the beast. Similarly, weight-for-age, weight-for-height and arm circumference each touch upon 'different aspects of the vague entity called malnutrition'; none gives us a view of the whole condition.

In the next chapter, we explore the adaptability view of malnutrition further by examining the scientific model of food requirements with which it is associated. The elephant analogy is again worth bearing in mind because it is a feature of all scientific models that they represent the phenomena being studied in a selective and deliberately simplified way. Only small parts of any elephant are adequately portrayed. In the physical sciences, the simplifications are obvious when investigators talk about 'ideal gases' or 'weightless bodies', or when they ignore friction. Useful conclusions can be drawn from such models, but when these conclusions are applied to the actual world, care and realism are needed.

The scientific view of malnutrition with which we are concerned simplifies and selects from the overall problem area by taking 'failure of function' as its basic criterion. Partly this is because physiological functions such as growth, or resistance to disease can be measured much more satisfactorily than, say, hunger: but also because we are making a judgement about the seriousness to individuals of the consequences of physiological break-down as compared to hunger, or minor forms of ill health. We must not forget that those value judgements have been made, and are implicit in every application of this (or any other) model.

Some comparable issues arise in connection with the so-called 'human capital' model of welfare policy discussed in Chapter 4. This represents a way of thinking about education and health services as 'investments' in human productive power, and as capable of being evaluated like other investments in cost-benefit terms. Such ideas may be of academic interest to economists, but could lead to very perverse decisions if applied without caution directly to policy. The same goes for biological concepts which regard the human body as a self-regulating machine. Either view might imply, for example, that welfare should be provided at a level which supports the maximum ratio of labour output to cost, regardless of whether the people who form the labour 'resource' experience hunger and distress. The models do not necessarily lead to such conclusions. They can be interpreted this way only if we forget that they are highly simplified views and do not represent the whole human condition.

It must be stressed, therefore, that the adaptability view of malnutrition and related scientific models are not intended to discount as unimportant the hunger and ill-health apparently associated with inadequate food intake. What they may do, however, is to encourage us to recognise circumstances where providing more and better food does not solve every problem. In many instances, for example, it will make more sense to improve water supplies or housing, to develop immunisation programmes or find ways of enabling mothers to devote more time to child care. More fundamentally, since the underlying reason why people have to put up with inadequate food and bad health is poverty, to over-state the case concerning malnutrition may distract governments from the politically uncomfortable task of redistributing wealth.

3 Energy and protein requirements*

Food energy estimates

Two kinds of statement are commonly made about the amount of food which people need. Firstly, figures are quoted for quantities of nutrients which could safely be recommended for practically all individuals, even though they may be living under a wide variety of situations. When energy is referred to, these figures are based on observed *average* intakes or expenditures in apparently healthy populations. Figures for other nutrients are for intakes which are adjusted according to the statistical distribution of individual measurements; they are set at two standard deviations above the average. These 'recommended intakes', or 'safe dietary allowances' are thus based on over-providing for the vast majority of people in order to ensure that everybody gets enough. Such a policy would certainly enable each individual to achieve his or her genetic potential for growth, and might be a sensible basis for planning diets for institutions. However, such figures are of little help in assessing the likelihood of malnutrition (Longhurst and Payne, 1979).

Secondly, however, estimates are sometimes quoted for minimum physiological requirements, that is, levels of intake below which there is an increasing probability that some

---

*This chapter is based mainly on material prepared by Philip Payne. See Payne, 1976, 1982.

specified symptom of deficiency will appear. The symptoms concerned are the failures of body function previously mentioned, such as growth in children, reproduction and work in adults, and failure to resist infection. Use of these criteria to define minimum requirements is, of course, consistent with the adaptability view of malnutrition discussed in the previous chapter, except that when figures are quoted, the extent to which requirements may vary with adaptation to different environments is not usually stated.

Most research has been done on western populations in which, for example, the pressure to follow a seasonal work pattern or to continue to work during pregnancy or lactation is relatively slight. Thus while we know something about levels of energy intake which on average are adequate for these populations, we know very little about populations which depend heavily on the seasonal use of stored energy and nutrients, or about populations adapted to a higher level of efficiency through small body size or in other ways.

Overall energy *expenditures* in the body depend on levels of activity, growth, body composition, diet and metabolic characteristics. All these are subject to adaptation, but the underlying rate of metabolism necessary for the *maintenance* of the functions of a resting individual is thought to be more consistent and predictable than most other factors. This is measured as the *basal metabolic rate* (BMR), and is found to vary with body weight in a fairly predictable way (Kleiber, 1961).

Because of this assumed regularity, and because BMR is clearly of fundamental importance, it was used by an FAO/WHO committee in 1971 as the starting point for their estimates of minimal energy requirements (FAO/WHO, 1973). However, the values of basal metabolic rate accepted by the committee referred to studies made on American subjects by Talbot (1938), and the measurements relate to resting but wakeful individuals who were comfortable and warm after an overnight fast of 12–15 hours. Metabolic rates *below* these accepted figures for the resting rate may in fact be recorded during sleep (Benedict, 1915); they may also be recorded in subjects who have adapted to a low food intake over a period of time or who are undisputably undernourished.

Table 3.1 *The effect of undernutrition on BMR; mean values reported from various studies*

Reference and number of subjects	Days of fast	Mean daily intake during fast		Percent change in BMR per person	Percent change in BMR per unit body weight
		MJ	kcal		
Benedict (1919) studying 24 subjects	120	5.85	1400	19	12
Beattie and Herbert (1947), 11 subjects	>100	<7.3	<1750	26	14
Keys *et al.* (1950), with 33 subjects	200	6.55	1570	39	19
Grande (1964)					
1 with 13 subjects	20	4.2	1000	17	9
2 with 12 subjects	14	4.2	1000	21	14

Observations of people undertaking partial fasts over long periods suggest that basal metabolic rates in underfed people may be anything between 10 and 30 per cent below the figures regarded as normal (Table 3.1; compare Kleitman, 1926). These observations would provide a rational explanation for the frequent reports that populations exist in developing countries which habitually consume extremely low food intakes without catastrophic results (Miller and Rivers, 1972; Norgan *et al.*, 1974).

It has been assumed that we can arrive at a figure for the food energy intake required to maintain body weight by working from BMR as a basis: hence the importance of measuring it. There are problems about doing so, however, of which the most serious is that we do not know the efficiency with which energy in food is converted and used by the body. Direct measurements of this efficiency in man are scarce. The FAO/WHO expert committee approached the problem by an ingenious comparative approach. As we have noted, BMR has a definite relationship with body weight that holds for most mammals as well as man. The FAO/WHO committee collated the evidence on food energy *intakes* at zero energy or zero nitrogen balance in experiments on animals and man; they showed that *this* too was related to body weight, and that it was consistently about 1.5 times greater than BMR. Thus they concluded that the minimal food energy cost of weight maintenance is approximately 1.5 × BMR.

This result could be used to estimate a minimum energy intake required to sustain life, and indeed was so used by FAO in its Fourth World Food Survey. FAO needed to take account of possible adaptations in body maintenance requirements and physiological efficiency which seem to allow some people to survive on less than 1.5 × BMR. Faced with this problem, FAO took the lower limit of normal variation of BMR (80 per cent of the mean value) and regarded it as a lower limit of adaptation. Hence they adopted a formula for the minimal energy cost of maintenance as 1.5 × 0.8 × BMR (= 1.2 BMR). FAO then accepted this value as a 'critical limit' for maintenance requirements which could be used in defining undernutrition.

The conventional method of analysing food energy requirements, according to Wood and Capstick (1928), partitions the energy expenditure of an animal into three separate components: maintenance, growth, and activity. These three components are assumed not to interact, and maintenance, which we have already considered, often represents the biggest part of the total energy demand. With regard to the energy cost of *growth*, the FAO/WHO committee estimated a requirement of 21KJ (5 kcal) above maintenance for every gramme of tissue gained. (This is in fact a high figure compared with some recorded values (e.g. Ashworth, 1969), but given the errors that must be involved in other parts of the food requirements estimate, accuracy with regard to this component matters little.)

The third component of energy expenditure is activity. Here, of course, the output of people doing manual work can be measured, and a typical figure of 0.735 MJ (175 kcal) per day for adults employed in agriculture is sometimes used as a basis for estimates (Bayliss-Smith, 1981). Bearing in mind the seasonality of agriculture, we may expect average work rates to be less than this. Peak demands may partly be met by drawing on body energy stores, so how much extra food is required to support his labour will depend on the efficiency of body storage as well as on the conversion efficiency of the muscles. Where people have adapted to a low food intake, that could partly be by increased efficiency, but probably also depends on a reduction in unnecessary exertion. There is evidence for both types of adaptation. Keys *et al.* (1950) reported that voluntary activity decreased during experimental semi-starvation, but also said that the energy cost of specified tasks was the same per unit of body weight throughout. This differs from Seckler's (1981) finding that overall work efficiency is inversely related to body weight over a limited range. But Keys agrees that the *total* energy cost of work tends to fall because body weight is reduced. Some physiologists have claimed that 'work capacity' is also impaired by undernutrition, but this is difficult to substantiate; in practice, the maximum rate of work a person can sustain is rarely important in limiting his or her effectiveness as a producer. Actual work rates are more often limited by the nature of the work itself, and by the social factors determining its organisation.

The outcome of all this is to leave maintenance as the dominant aspect of food energy requirements, especially for people surviving on very low intakes. Thus FAO equated their estimate of minimum maintenance requirement with the minimum energy intake required to sustain life. So we end up with two different kinds of estimate for human energy requirements, one an observed average and the other an estimated minimum, the latter being intended to represent a 'critical limit' of adaptation to low food intakes.

To illustrate the difference between these two kinds of requirement, we may consider the energy needs of a 'reference man', aged 25 to 40 and weighing 65 kg. The figures are as follows:

1. recommended intake (FAO/WHO, 1973), equivalent to a predicted average intake for a well-fed population: 12.5 MJ/day (3000 kcal/day);
2. minimum physiological needs, corresponding to a critical limit of adaptation taken as 1.2 BMR (FAO, 1977): 7.5 MJ/day (1800 kcal/day).

The corresponding figures for a 55 kg woman of the same age who is neither pregnant nor lactating are 9.2 and 6.3 MJ/day (2200 and 1500 kcal/day).

Neither figure, of course, can be regarded as a correct statement of the requirements of any specific group of real human beings. The higher figure is now generally thought to over-estimate requirements in most populations. As to the lower figure, this refers to people who are likely to be experiencing hunger, often painfully and for long periods, but whose essential body functions are not impaired. We have noted some of the arbitrary assumptions in its estimation, and have pointed out that to quote a single figure ignores the variations to be expected in different environments. Lipton (1982) stresses that a lower limit of energy intake will not only vary between individuals, gene pools, age-groups, and so on, but that it also depends on the choices people make (or are forced to make) about maintaining work output when food is short. We may well end up by questioning whether it can ever make sense to state requirements in this way, rather than specifying ranges, or stating them relative to local conditions.

It is worth recalling the three apparently healthy populations with sharply contrasting lifestyles which were referred to in Tables 1.1 and 1.2. Body weights in these populations were mostly less than for the reference man and woman quoted above, but the range of average intakes for the groups represented is from 8.12 to 14.4 MJ/day for men, and from 5.94 to 12.1 MJ/day for women, varying with season.

Adaptations and responses

The foregoing discussion left many questions unanswered about the energy required for work in populations surviving on very low intakes. Two factors need to be considered: long-term *adaptations*, particularly in body size, and short-term *responses* to temporary (or seasonal) food shortages. The latter include physiological responses whereby the conversion efficiency of energy in the body can rise when intakes fall. This may happen, for example, if food energy is used directly as glucose instead of being converted to fat and released at some later time, and other variations in the pathways for energy use may take place. But behavioural responses to reduced intake are important also, and Lipton (1982, p.36) pointedly asks: 'Suppose a body *can*, when daily intake falls 10 per cent, maintain work levels and cut requirements via higher conversion efficiency. To what extent will different groups of people choose not to reduce work...so forcing their bodies to "raise conversion efficiency"?' Nothing is known about such matters.

With regard to long-term adaptation, one necessary adjustment in conventional thinking concerns the status of individuals who are small and under-weight by international standards, but who show no signs of functional impairment. The nutritional status of such people has often been described as 'mild malnutrition' when populations are screened by height or by weight in relation to age, but it might be better to regard them as 'small but healthy' where no contrary evidence exists. The latter interpretation may seem especially relevant in the light of what has already been said about adaptations to a wide range of seasonal and work environments. Before people are classed as malnourished, therefore, and before their food intakes are deemed insufficient, we ought to examine the environments from which such people have come, and consider the question of adaptation.

For example, traditional diets in Japan have produced many small but undoubtedly fit people. With current trends to more westernised eating habits, many individuals are growing taller and heavier, but there is concern that they may be more vulnerable to the degenerative diseases of later life, and that stamina for work may be less. Certainly there are no objective data to support the idea that western diets and western anthropometric standards represent an optimum.

Under conditions of food scarcity, in particular, there may be distinct advantages in small body size, since nutrient requirements are related to body weight. However, Gopalan (1983) and others have advanced a strong argument against this position. Since large people have more muscle tissue than small people, their work capacity is greater and therefore they can earn more in manual labour than small people. A commonly cited study in support of this position is that of Satyanarayana *et al.* (1977) showing that among 47 workers engaged in assembling fuses into bundles on a piecework wage basis, the heavier workers consistently produced more than the lighter workers even in this moderate level of work activity.

Seckler (1981) argues that we should not confuse total production with efficient use of energy in production. Although the heavier workers produced more, they may have done so less efficiently. Two contrary points should be noted, however. Firstly, this job was paid as piecework, which may have led to untypical results. Secondly, it was light industrial work for which the energy requirements of people when they were on the job would be dominated by body maintenance needs rather than muscular energy expenditures. In these latter conditions, it is certainly likely that small people would be more efficient.

In heavy work, there is no evidence of any particular body size favouring high efficiency; muscular energy conversion efficiency is now thought to be the most important rate limiting step and this is not likely to be affected by body size. In studies of road workers made by Tandon *et al.* (1975), the bigger, heavier men certainly tended to produce a greater work output. But in a comparison of those with the highest outputs and those with the lowest, food energy intakes were found to be almost the same. When local workers (average body weight 45.5 kg) were compared with group of more practised road workers from outside the area (average weight 50.4 kg), it was found that the latter did more work with a lower food energy intake. Their efficiency in this respect was about 50 per cent greater, apparently due mainly to their greater experience and dexterity.

With regard to heavy manual work, therefore, small people do not seem to have any advantage, but it does seem possible that populations of 'small but healthy' people represent other kinds of adaptation with respect to work and survival; especially because for them, maintenance requirements are less. What we need to notice, however, is that small body size is an adaptation which is made during growth, sometimes at the cost of considerable deprivation. By contrast, we have also talked about short-term modifications of behaviour and metabolism related to seasonal conditions, describing these as 'responses' to low food intakes. They are sustained for a few months at most, and where they entail the depletion of body stores of fat or nutrients, they are clearly not sustainable in the long term.

This distinction between sustained adaptation and short-term response is important if 'critical limits of adaptation' are specified for use in assessing the extent of undernutrition in a population. In most circumstances, we will be enquiring whether people's capacity for short-term response is overstretched, and we will be assuming that any long-term adaptations are fixed. But such adaptations must differ markedly from one region and one social group to another, and the limits of response within that long-term framework must presumably also differ. Thus even if the critical limit of 1.2 BMR is a reasonable best estimate of the lowest level to which existing social groups will be found to have adapted, it should not be regarded as a limit below which no further adaptation is possible.

Some of these ideas challenge the conventional wisdom about the *variability* of human food requirements. They conflict with the belief that each individual in a population has his or her own specific requirement level for energy or protein, related to genetic potential for growth and health, and in some way fixed for that individual. People are acknowledged to differ slightly, but in a way that is assumed to conform with a normal Gaussian distribution. Standard deviation is then a clear and unambiguous expression of the extent of variations.

By contrast, the arguments put forward in this chapter imply that individuals each have a range of possible responses appropriate to a range of food intakes, and are not characterised by any fixed requirement. Indeed, Sukhatme has argued that the very notion of a fixed requirement is in conflict with most of the evidence collected over the last forty years. The data are much more satisfactorily understood in terms of a self-regulating, homeostatic model (Sukhatme and Margen, 1978).

This is a complex idea, but a simple analogy may be useful in showing what it involves. Suppose a leaking bucket is being filled at a pump. It is possible to adjust the flow into the bucket so that it exactly matches the rate of leakage. Then equilibrium is maintained, with a steady water level. We can alter the rate of inflow so that equilibrium is reached with the bucket almost full, or with the bucket nearly empty. In the latter case, the rate of leakage is less because of lower pressure, and perhaps because some leaks are above the water line; thus a lower rate of inflow is necessary. Clearly, there is a range of flows over which many different equilibrium states are possible. There is also a critical lower limit of inflow below which the bucket empties, and an upper limit, beyond which it overflows. To some extent, at least, the responses of the human body to variations in food intake are similar.

One implication is that when we observe a range of different food intakes in an apparently healthy population, this not only reflects variability between individuals, but more fundamentally, it reflects a range of possible equilibrium states for each of those people. Thus standard deviation takes on a different significance, since it is now seen to represent the potential for *response* to changes, rather than random statistical differences. A food intake that is below average by a matter of two standard deviations conventionally represents an intake which is lower than the requirements of all but 2.5 per cent of the population; according to Sukhatme however it could just as reasonably be taken as an estimate of the lower limit of possible adapted responses in that population.

Applied to food energy intakes, this estimate gives a rather low figure for minimum physiological requirements, but not as low as that obtained from FAO's (1977) assumption that the lower limit of adaptation for many populations might be around 1.2 BMR. For example, working on two standard deviations below the average, Sukhatme (1961) calculated the minimum for a 55 kg man as 8.8 MJ or 2100 kcal, which is 22 per cent below the FAO/WHO recommended intake, whereas using $1.2 \times$ BMR gives a value of 40 per cent below.

This example of extremes reinforces the warnings about scientific models that were sounded at the end of Chapter 2, since in this instance, one's choice of model affects conclusions very substantially. In fact little has been done in a systematic way to test the various models. A major difficulty is that knowledge of adult human requirements is largely based on experiments in which the objective has been to maintain equilibrium. The argument applies to protein as well as to energy intakes, and experiments have been done on apparently healthy people in which levels of intake are found which are just sufficient to maintain the existing level of body nitrogen. However, the assumption then made that nitrogen balance indicates adequate intake is not valid. It is, rather, just an indicator that the subject's equilibrium state is not changing; the significance for health of the changes in equilibrium state that do commonly occur is not known.

Even if the adaptability model comes to be accepted as being closer to reality than that currently advocated by FAO and WHO committees, it will still not provide us with a completely general basis for prediction because of other factors which influence variability. Measurements made at a single point in time on individuals of the same age and sex will include at least the following sources of variance:

1. differences in *adaptation*, including those reflecting the primary expression of genetic factors, and those arising from the effects of diet and environment during growth;
2. differences due to the extent and nature of continuous auto-regulatory *responses*;
3. a 'noise' component due to random, unrelated fluctuation in the environment, or diet, or due to measurement errors.

If we were to conduct experiments in order to establish the safe limits of adaptive response to different intakes of some nutrients, we would need to distinguish between these sources of variability. Assuming that in general we would find both upper and lower limits to the range, with some risk of dysfunction attached to high levels of intake as well as low levels, the situation would be as shown in the diagram (Figure 3.1). Instead of a single figure for the recommended intake or safe level for the particular nutrient, we would have a 'safe range', with upper and lower limits bounded by points for which the probability of dysfunction rises above an acceptable level.

'Adaptive' models of body weight control

The concept of an adaptive, self-regulating system implies some type of negative feedback response by which the body is able in part to cancel out changes in inputs and outputs, and maintain the internal state near its original condition. There will be several such feedback loops, and in the particular case of energy, one even extends outside the body, so that an individual may adapt by modifying his interaction with the environment, and hence change his requirements for energy to bring them into line with

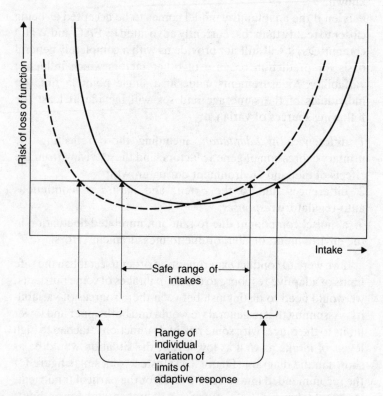

Figure 3.1   Schematic view of the range of adaptive responses likely to be encountered with different levels of nutrient intake

intake. Thus the total strategy of adaptive response for energy comprises individual and social changes in behaviour as well as changes in body weight, body composition and metabolic regulation. It may well be that individuals differ in the relative balance of these components, and that for some, changes in behaviour will be a more important adaptive mechanism than for others.

On a physiological level, it is clear that individuals differ very markedly with regard to energy storage within the body. For the majority, energy is chiefly stored in the form of fat, but for a few people, significant quantitites of energy are also stored as protein. We can represent these differences by defining a ratio which represents the proportion of energy stored as protein in the body. The same ratio predicts the energy mobilized from protein when energy intake is less than expenditure. The 'P-value' (Payne and Dugdale, 1977) expresses this component of energy as a ratio of the total energy stored in the form of fat and lean tissues in the body (or the total energy mobilised when intakes fall). Figure 3.2 shows the proportions of energy mobilised from protein in semi-starving men as observed by Keys *et al.* (1950), and it is evident that these men showed a wide variation in the way they responded to a negative energy balance. On average, 15 per cent of energy was lost from lean tissue stores and 85 per cent from fat. But the average actually spans a tenfold range: some individuals lost only 3 per cent of energy from protein, others as much as 30 per cent.

We do not know the extent to which the propensity to store and utilise protein as opposed to fat is a result of genetic differences, and how much is a result of patterns established during early growth. We do know that under some circumstances, a tendency to use fat as an energy store might be a good survival strategy, whereas in other circumstances it could lead to obesity. The nature of responses to increased energy intakes may be similarly varied. The data of Miller and Mumford (1967) showed considerable variations between individuals in respect of degree of weight gain during overfeeding. This may partly be because the metabolic efficiency of energy storage varies from one person to another and partly because some people are less

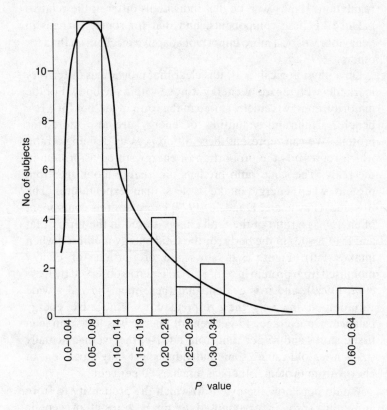

$$P = \left(\frac{\text{energy stored as, or mobilised from protein}}{\text{total energy stored in the body, or mobilised}} \right)$$

Figure 3.2   Differences between individual men with respect to the storage of energy as fat or as protein

Notes: P-value would be zero for an individual whose body store of energy consisted solely of fat, and 1.0 for an individual storing energy solely as protein.

Source: Dugdale and Payne 1977, based on data from the experiments of Keys *et al.* 1950.

efficient when they over eat. It also seems likely that individuals with a propensity for fat storage will gain more weight before increased metabolism balances out the higher intake than will individuals who store metabolically active lean tissue.

Protein requirements

As we know so little about the complex strategy of response and adaptation, and have no reliable indicators to predict how a given individual will respond to changes in intake, either by body weight, composition, or behaviour, the definition of energy requirements is an uncertain business. In respect of protein, we are hardly better off. Obsession with nitrogen balance as a 'criterion' of adequacy has led to a neglect of the study of adaptive changes and mechanisms. Nonetheless, it is well established that such mechanisms exist. Waterlow (1981) has reviewed the evidence for adaptive responses in nitrogen metabolism, and concluded that the body possesses powerful mechanisms for economising on nitrogen.

For example, Durkin *et al.* (1981) showed that in most cases, responses to reduced levels of nitrogen intake included the loss of body weight, Nicol and Phillips (1976) showed that Nigerian farmers, habituated to diets relatively low in protein, utilised that protein more efficiently than American subjects, and could maintain balance on about 30 per cent less. It appears that the Nigerians were adapted to low intake.

Considering that little is known about such adaptations, it is not surprising that efforts to define human protein requirements have had a chequered history. 'Kwashiorkor' was described by Williams (1933) as an illness, 'in which some amino acid or protein deficiency cannot be excluded'. The children who developed the disease did so after weaning, when they were fed on starchy porridge rather low in protein, energy and other nutrients, and they were cured by milk. In time, the idea that this syndrome was specifically caused by protein deficiency became generally established.

Subsequent work, however, challenged the definition of kwashiorkor as protein deficiency, and has led to a revision of ideas about how much protein young children need. Lower values for their protein requirements have slowly gained acceptance, but energy needs are still estimated to be at around the same level (Table 3.2). No set of symptoms or signs is now generally agreed to be evidence of a specific deficiency of *protein* in man. This is, of course, not to say that there is no malnutrition in children, nor is it to deny that there is such a thing as kwashiorkor. It is simply that neither clinical studies nor attempts to reproduce the condition in animals provide sufficient justification for identifying the well-known symptoms (oedema, hair and skin changes, fatty liver, blood changes) as specific for protein or amino acid deficiency (Waterlow and Payne, 1975).

The results of food consumption measurements made on individual children in a variety of societies seem to confirm this conclusion (Waterlow and Rutishauser, 1974). Where intakes of protein are low relative to estimates of requirements, so also are intakes of energy, and often all other essential nutrients as well. But these deficits of nutrients are often such as would be made

Table 3.2   *Estimates of protein and energy requirements at 1 year of age, corresponding to 'recommended intakes'*

Year	Per kg body weight			Ratio of protein energy to total energy %	Source
	Protein[1] g	Energy MJ	kcal		
1948	3.3	0.42	100	13.2	NAS (1948)[2]
1957	2.0	0.42	100	8.0	FAO (1957)
1963	2.5	0.42	100	10.0	NAS (1963)[2]
1965	1.1	0.42	100	4.4	FAO/WHO (1965)
1968	1.8	0.42	100	7.2	NAS (1968)[2]
1969	1.3	0.47	110	4.7	DHSS (1969)[3]
1973	1.25	0.44	105	4.8	FAO/WHO (1973)
1974	1.35	0.42	100	5.4	NAS (1974)[3]

[1] As protein which is 100% utilised.
[2] US source; protein estimates consistently higher than in other sources.
[3] UK source.

good automatically if energy needs were satisifed by taking more of the same food. Thus the most significant factor causing child malnutrition would seem to be simply inadequate food intake.

Because of their rapid growth rates, infants need a somewhat higher proportion of protein in their diets than is required by older children and young adults. But we need to remember that protein plays a highly complex role in physiology. It is at once a nutrient in its own right, and a source of energy. When protein levels in diets are high, a large proportion of the amino acids derived from protein is deaminated and oxidised as fuel. This also occurs in situations of overall energy deficit. Thus a child given an adequate protein diet, but at intake levels below his or her energy needs, will not derive full benefit for growth from the protein, but will use it as an energy source.

A further complication is that proteins do not all have the same growth-promoting value. Depending on the balance of their component amino acids, some have higher 'quality' than others. Protein quality indexes (such as 'net protein utilisation', or 'chemical score') are estimates of the percentage of the total protein which can be expected to be utilised for growth and maintenance in a young animal or a child. On this basis, eggs and milk have efficiencies close to 100 per cent. A food or diet with a quality of 70 per cent will contribute more of its amino acids to growth than one of 40 per cent. However, the amino acids which are not used for protein metabolism will not be wasted: rather, they will be diverted for use as an energy source.

Because protein can provide the body with energy in this way, at roughly 17 KJ or 4 kcal from each gramme converted, it is useful and usual to express the protein value of diets in relation to their energy content. The relevant ratio, expressed as a *percentage*, is given by one of the following formulae, depending on the units employed:

$$\text{protein-energy ratio} = \frac{(\text{grammes protein in diet} \times 0.017 \times 100)}{\text{total megajoules in diet}}$$

$$= \frac{(\text{grammes protein in diet} \times 4 \times 100)}{\text{total kilocalories in diet}}$$

A further refinement is possible by correcting the energy value of the proteins by a factor which takes quality into account. The result is a ratio of energy derived from fully utilisable protein: the 'net dietary protein-energy ratio' (NDpE%) (Payne, 1972).

Animals are often used to assess the nutritional values of different foods, and for example to compare different strains and varieties of cereal grains as protein sources. Thus the superior growth of rats and pigs on high lysine varieties of maize and rice have often been cited as evidence of their advantages for humans. However, in interpreting such feeding trials it is important to note the major differences that exist in the nutrient needs of different species.

Most young mammals grow very much faster than human infants when growth is measured as weight gain per unit body weight, and need a larger proportion of protein in the diets to support this growth. Figure 3.3 illustrates the point diagramatically. If feeding experiments were carried out with an adult man, a one-year-old child, a new-born baby, and a young pig, using a diet containing 10 per cent of a protein, one of whose amino acids could be varied from zero up to 100 per cent (with perfect balance of all other amino

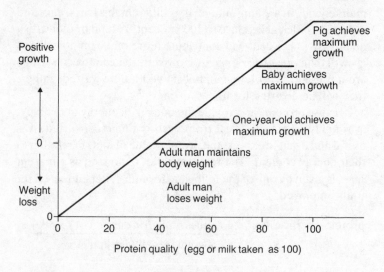

Figure 3.3   Feeding experiments based on a diet containing 10 per cent protein of varying quality

acids), then the man would lose weight with a zero ratio, and would show improvement as the level was raised up to about 40 per cent of maximum, and then no further response. Similarly, the one-year-old would continue to benefit from increases up to about 50 per cent, the new-born baby up to 70–80 per cent, but the pig up to 100 per cent.

It should be stressed that this diagram represents the protein requirements for maximum growth in human babies, which is not the same thing as the optimum protein requirement. Children, unlike pigs, are not deliberately fattened for market, so it should not be assumed that the fastest rate of growth is necessarily the best; indeed, we will shortly quote reasons for thinking that it is not. What the diagram makes clear, however, is that the growth of children does not always suffer if protein quality is less than 100. In any practical situation, what has to be assessed is whether the quantity of protein eaten, in conjunction with the balance of amino acids, i.e. its quality, is such that the requirements of the consumer for the most limiting amino acid are met. The balance of evidence from feeding trials seems to show that although cereals are limited in protein quality by their content of lysine, threonine and tryptophan, and although this is as true for children as it is for pigs, provided that sufficient cereal is consumed to meet energy and total protein needs, then conventional varieties of most cereals contain sufficient of these amino acids to meet the requirements even of preschool children.

As with energy, so with protein, therefore, the conclusion to emerge from this chapter is that human food requirements are less certainly known than was once thought. This ought not to be regarded as totally discouraging, however, but rather as a challenge to regard nutrition with a more comprehensive understanding of physiological function and environmental constraint. Part of that challenge is to combine these insights with a study of the variability between individuals' capacity to adapt to environmental changes without unacceptable loss of function. Up to now, many nutritionists have tended to overlook this problem area, partly because of the difficulty of studying it experimentally, but partly also because the models conventionally used to describe the interaction of requirements and nutrient intake implicitly assume that under normal conditions, adaptation is a relatively minor part of total variability. If adaptation does occur, the assumption has usually been that the situation must be abnormal, and failing proof to the contrary, the adapted state is regarded as likely to confer some disadvantage.

Conclusions

When a nutritional requirement level is stated, a prediction is being made on the basis of past knowledge about the probability of specific functional disabilities affecting a particular group or individual. Ideally, the requirement level should be presented in a form which indicates this fact. However, it has to be admitted that few satisfactory statements of this kind are possible, e.g. that 'there is a probability of 0.1 ± 0.01 that fifteen-year-old non-pregnant females will develop night blindness if they sustain an intake of less than 400 RE (retinal equivalents) of vitamin A per day' (needless to say, we do not know if this is in fact true). Ideally, too, the probability should be established within confidence limits, and the dysfunction to which it refers should be specified and measurable. Other kinds of dysfunction related to vitamin A status may be known to exist, and their probabilities could also be stated for that sample level of intake. Since many dysfunctions have multiple causes, some statement about the context (environment infection, etc.) might also be necessary. Where other departures from health may only be suspected, no true requirement figure can or should be stated with respect to these.

Something which is specifically excluded from this definition is the notion of an 'optimum' state of nutritional health, achievement of which might be the criterion for a requirement level. This is an idealistic notion which seems to be sustained by two kinds of attitude. One is a view which reacts against minimum prescriptions, and would prefer to see emphasis placed on the complete fulfilment of human genetic potential. This feeling demands respect, and if resources were available – and if the concept of genetic potential could be clarified – policies based on such ideas would deserve support.

The other attitude is that optimum states are somehow inherent in 'natural' systems, and that the right nutritional conditions are those that allow these states to be expressed. This is commonly linked to the idea that natural selection will have maximised 'fitness', and that there should exist a state of nutrition in the individual which will be a reflection of that fitness. However, we have no reason to believe that there is some preferred state of metabolism or physiology in the individual which simultaneously brings to a maximum all qualities that we happen to consider desirable, and so, at the other end of life, is longevity. But there is no evolutionary selection for longevity – only for survival to sexual maturity (Kirkwood, 1977). Nor is there any evidence that children who grow rapidly enjoy long life. Indeed, to the extent that experiments with animals can throw light on the matter, Ross *et al.* (1976) found that when young rats were allowed to select their own diets, there was considerable individual variation in food energy consumption and growth rate, and that high rates were negatively correlated with lifespan. In this instance, at least, it is clear that energy requirements for young animals could be based either on the criterion of achieving the full genetic potential for early growth, or on subsequent longevity, but not both.

Whether or not this evidence can be paralleled in humans, it serves by analogy to show why any views of 'desirable' or 'optimal' food intakes for human individuals or groups can only be value judgements. If our aim is to be as objective as possible, we have to be content with describing how the probability of failure to sustain function varies with intake. Deciding what levels of probability or risk are unacceptable, brings us back to value statements again. What is quite clear is that where energy and protein requirements are concerned, doing this leads to critical limits considerably below what many people would judge to be desirable.

Yet science is not objective and value-free. The preceding paragraph is itself a value-judgement above the limits of the scientist's responsibilities. Other aspects of the value-system inherent in science are reflected in the simplifications which scientists build into their models, and are to be observed also in uncritical reverence for measurements and statistics. This is often exploited by policy-makers who use the figures so produced both to legitimise past actions and to guide their plans. Enough has been said here to stress that our understanding of individual adaptability with regard to food is extremely sparse. That clearly limits our ability to make quantitative statements about nutrient requirements. Yet over the years, governments and international agencies have produced a stream of reports listing minimum physiological requirements, safe levels, and recommended dietary allowances, which are supposed to have a firm objective basis. In subsequent chapters, we shall describe an approach to the use of quantitative data which we believe can be much more helpful in understanding malnutrition and in informing action to reduce its incidence.

4   Food system indicators*

Variables in food systems

Two kinds of measurement used in monitoring food systems have
been discussed in previous pages: anthropometric assessments of
nutritional status (Chapter 2), and measurements of food intake
related to ideas about requirements (Chapter 3). In considering
food supply and utilisation over a whole nation, as well as the
nutritional status of its people, there are obviously many other
variables which might usefully be measured: food stocks and
production, for example, or people's expenditure on food. Figure
4.1 is developed from the food system diagram presented earlier
(Figure 1.1) in order to show whereabouts in the system observations are commonly made or data collected. All the variables
concerned are examples of *system variables*. The values they take at
any one moment reflect the *state of the system* at that moment.
Normally, a variety of processes and changes will be continuously
under way, and measurements of these variables specify the state of
the system in 'frozen' form, rather like photographs taken at
particular instants.

It will be noticed that these system variables are of two kinds.
Some, like body weight or food stocks, are characteristic of a

---

*This chapter is based on material prepared by Peter Cutler, Elizabeth Dowler,
Philip Payne, Young Ok Seo, Anne Thomson and Erica Wheeler. Fuller versions of
some of the material have been published by Dowler *et al.*, (1982) and also by
Dowler and Seo (1983).

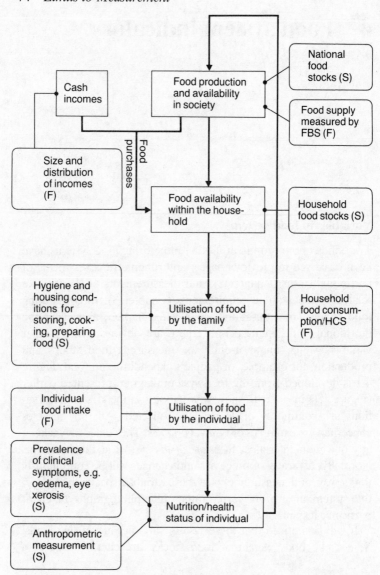

Figure 4.1   The food system of a region or nation as it was defined in Chapter 1, but now showing some of the system variables which are commonly measured
Notes: F denotes variables which measure flows through the system; S denotes variables which reflect conditions within the system.

condition in the system that is liable to change fairly slowly. Others measure flows through the system, and like the flow from a tap, they can fluctuate widely or even be abruptly turned off. One example is cash income, which drops to zero overnight when an individual loses his job. Clearly, these two kinds of variable reflect on the state of the system in different ways. Much confusion surrounding data on energy or protein intakes arises because these latter are flows, yet some people insist on treating the figures as if they represent an established condition of either adequate or inadequate nutrition. The distinction can be understood by referring again to a leaking bucket that is being filled at a pump. Measuring the flow of water from the pump cannot tell us how full the bucket is – we have to observe or measure that directly.

The interpretation of measurements often involves checking them against critical levels of the variables to which they refer. These are levels below (or above) which it is generally agreed there is evidence of an unacceptable degree of immediate or impending distress. It is essentially the use of cut-off points defining such levels which distinguishes the particular variables which we choose to define as *indicators*, from other system variables.

The levels at which cut-off points are set should ideally depend on the purpose for which the indicator is being used. We have seen how this works for anthropometric measurements, where a working definition of a cut-off point for, say, weight-for-age, is defined to fit particular circumstances, and may vary according to whether the purpose is surveillance or screening. With regard to food intakes, the critical points are the requirement figures and estimates of adaptability limits, and which ones we use may again depend on our purpose. If the aim is to identify social groups with the most seriously inadequate diets, we might use an estimate for the lower critical limit of adaptation. If, however, the aim is to buy sufficient food for residents in an institution, we would certainly use a higher requirement figure.

To sum up, then, an indicator is a variable such as food intake or weight-for-age for which critical points have been agreed. A simple example from outside our subject is provided by the gauge which indicates steam pressure in a boiler. Here, the 'system', or set of components, consists of boiler, fire-box and engine. Steam pressure is the system variable which we select to describe the state of that system. In addition to measuring pressure, the steam gauge may also have certain critical points marked on the pressure scale, below which pressure is inadequate, or above which is a danger of explosion. It is these critical points which make steam pressure an indicator of the state of the boiler.

A normal characteristic of an indicator is that it is used to show a number of different aspects of the performance of a system. In this example, the situation is relatively simple because steam pressure is quantitatively related in a known way to other variables such as temperature, and strain in the walls of the boiler. Steam pressure also tells us about the balance between steam output from the boiler and fuel input, but it does not allow us to estimate these flows directly.

In an instance like this, where the relationship between variables is unambiguous and clear, we may use one variable as a 'shorthand' indicator of another without hesitation. In biological and social systems, however, matters are rarely so simple. We may know that, within a particular kind of system, certain variables have usually assumed values which bear consistent mathematical relationships with each other, but we may not know how this happens. In such circumstances, a variable may not have a sufficiently well defined significance to be regarded as a shorthand indicator, but it might be generally accepted as a *proxy* for a set of system variables, or even for certain aspects of the system which cannot as yet be precisely defined.

Nutritional indicators based on anthropometry are to some extent *shorthand indicators*, when weight and size are taken as estimates of body nutrient stores, and size at a given age is regarded as a measure of the previous pattern of growth. But in addition, anthropometric indicators are commonly used as *proxies* for 'nutritional status', an imprecise notion that, as we have seen, covers the outcomes of a wide range of different processes, including the effects of different nutrient deficiencies, and of non-nutritional factors such as infection.

Defining the critical points which are associated with the use of indicators must always involve the expression of *value judgements*, and attempts to achieve consensus about acceptable levels of risk.

With regard to the boiler, for example, the owner of the plant may see advantages in terms of efficiency in running it at a high steam pressure, and provided he can afford the insurance premium, he may be happy to accept an increased risk of explosion. The men who stoke the boiler, however, may see no advantage in the higher pressure, but will be aware of a greater risk of injury or death. Their trade union might seek a much more stringent standard of safety than the management wishes to accept.

This illustrates a question which was raised in previous chapters but has not so far been answered. When we define malnutrition in terms of unacceptable levels of dysfunction, who decides what is unacceptable? The scientist cannot do this alone, despite the fact that he or she possesses some of the necessary information. With regard to the boiler, for example, an engineer might be called in to advise, but is in no position to judge what insurance premium the firm can afford, nor what level of risk the stokers (and their families) are willing to accept. Thus the engineer has to explore with the management, or perhaps with the trade union, what would be the consequences for them of a higher steam pressure and a greater risk. In other words, valuations of risk and of what is acceptable or otherwise should arise from a process of dialogue, either explicit or indirect, in which the scientist or technician is only one of the parties involved.

In nutrition, as in other fields, the role of the scientist is defined partly by his or her expertise in using a range of specialised techniques for observation, measurement and prediction. However, in no sense is his or her responsibility limited to this. Besides the work of measurement there are questions of social valuation, and whereas the former is a purely technical activity, the latter entails dialogue in some form with other sectors of society – with planners, no doubt, with those who fund research, and also, we might hope, with the ultimate consumers of the food. One of the differences between measuring a variable and using an indicator is that the former is a more or less objective technical activity while the latter always involves the use of critical points which express social valuations.

Indicators commonly used

We have already commented on the use of anthropometric indicators in the food system. We will now look at two other sets of indicators commonly used: food supply and consumption, and expenditure on food items.

Food supply and consumption

Among the more important variables that reflect on the operation of food systems are data on food supplies collected at national level, which are commonly expressed as per capita protein or energy availability. Such data are based on national food balance sheets (FBS) compiled regularly for many countries in a manner that takes account of food production, imports, exports and increases or decreases in food stocks. Grain used for seed or animal feed is subtracted, and so are estimated losses. (For detailed accounts of methodology, see FAO, 1980; Poleman, 1981.)

Despite several decades of effort, errors in these estimates are still known to be significant, and some authors suggest that for low income countries especially, they tend towards the understatement of food available (Poleman, 1981). Figures expressed as per caput supply introduce additional errors wherever population data are inaccurate. Moreover, as the food system diagram emphasises (Figure 4.1), FBS data represent flows through the system at a point which is rather remote from the individual eating a meal. Thus the figures do not represent human consumption, nor do they represent food distribution over time or over population. With good reason, the FAO cautions against misunderstanding their basis (FAO, 1980).

The usual way of estimating actual food intakes is through household consumption surveys (HCS, Figure 4.1). These employ a range of methods including weighed intake surveys (larder stocks or plate/pot consumption), diary recording and recall interviews (Marr, 1971; Burk and Pao, 1976, 1980).

Among the difficulties involved in using this method are problems of sampling and of seasonality in food supply or usage.

A further problem is that precise methods of weighing meals or ingredients tend to be intrusive, and may induce behavioural change and untypical intakes. Variation in eating patterns from day to day compound the problem, and household-based measurements usually omit food eaten outside the home, although in some instances, an estimate of food and/or nutrients in this category is included when results are published.

Do these two sources of data on food give the same information? Since FBS and HCS measurements of per capita food flows are made at different points in the system, we would not expect them to yield precisely the same results. Furthermore, FBS estimates cover 356 days; while HCS measurements typically cover 3–7 day periods in each household. Yet the differences which do occur have proved difficult to explain. FBS figures are always greater by about 1 MJ per capita in less developed countries, and by 3–4 MJ per capita in developed regions.

These differences may arise partly because alcohol and casually gathered fruit and nuts are not always included in the surveys as 'food'. Such mismatching cannot account for the discrepancies fully, however. Much emphasis is placed by some authorities on underestimation of wastage in the home as a source of error in HCS data in developed countries, but studies in Britain have failed to demonstrate such underestimation (Dowler, 1977; Wenlock *et al.*, 1977, 1980).

In Japan, a nationwide survey of household food consumption based on seven-day weighed intakes has been carried out annually for over thirty years, and an interesting comparison can be made between HCS and FBS figures over the whole of that period (Seo, 1981). Figure 4.2 shows the results graphically, plotted against per caput gross national product (GNP) on a log scale. Average energy intake as measured by HCS remains reasonably constant over the period considered. However, per caput energy supply as judged by FBS figures rose rapidly as GNP increased. Comparison with cross-sectional data from other countries shows that not only is the FBS estimate always higher than the household estimate, but the discrepancy increases as the economy of a country, and thus its food system, becomes more extensive and complex, with more opportunities

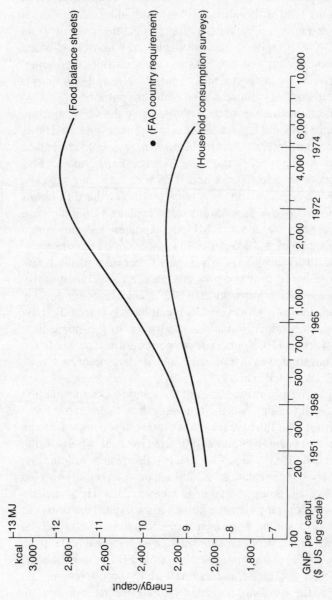

Figure 4.2 Longitudinal comparison – Japan (energy and GNP/caput: energy supply data (food balance sheets) and energy intake data (household consumption surveys))

Source: Seo 1981.

for loss or waste within the system as a whole, before reaching the household level.

Given the difficulties associated with these food supply data, and the uncertainty in estimates of 'requirements', efforts to use FBS figures to identify countries with an 'energy deficit' are bound to run into difficulties. Yet official bodies continue to describe global and national energy deficits in this way. The US Department of Agriculture produced two *World Food Budgets* relating to the 1960s (USDA, 1961, 1964) which concluded that almost the entire population of the developing world lived in 'diet deficient' countries. The World Bank (1976), using data from the 1960s, saw a problem of roughly the same magnitude involving about 1200 million people; or some 60–70 per cent of the total population of the countries represented. FAO has tried to modify FBS to estimate intakes by imposing an apparent distribution on the mean figure; this process leads to an estimated total number of people affected by 'protein energy malnutrition' of just over 400 million (FAO, 1974, 1977).

When FBS data are used to produce figures of this latter sort, what has happened is that the *system variable* measured by food balance sheets has been turned into an *indicator* by the application of a cut-off point. This latter is either a minimum level of food consumption or a recommended intake adjusted for such characteristics of the local population as age structure or average body weight (as in FAO's 'country requirement' figures).

Expenditure on food items

Since purchases of food intervene between the points in the food system where FBS and HCS measurements are taken (Figure 4.1), it might seem that a further way of exploring the operation of this part of the system might be to enquire into family food expenditures. As usual, there are several difficulties to be overcome. Spending on food by low income families as quoted to survey teams is quite often greater than the reported income of the same families; the former is over-estimated and/or the latter is under-reported (Scott and Mathew, 1983). In addition, there is little agreement about how data on family income should be

used. Again we are turning a system variable into an indicator by
defining some particular low income as a cut-off point, which
then becomes a 'poverty line'. But as we saw with the indicators
previously discussed, unless the cut-off point is carefully defined
in relation to some clear, practical purpose, its use may be
misleading.

With indicators derived from anthropometry, we have seen
cut-off points can be set at levels at which specified risks of
physiological dysfunction begin to rise steeply. An attempt to
introduce similar 'objective' criteria into the definition of a
poverty line has been made by Lipton (1982). He notes that the
poorest people in a wide range of countries commonly spend an
irreducible 20 per cent of their income on non-food essentials.
He further takes account of the tendency of food requirements
figures to over-estimate food needs, especially in relation to
'small but healthy' people living in warm climates, and with
Sukhatme's (1961) work in mind, he suggests that it might be
more realistic to work with 80 per cent of the conventional
requirements figures. This leads him to a 'double 80' rule,
according to which people are judged to be 'ultra poor' if 80 per
cent of their income is insufficient to purchase 80 per cent of
conventionally defined food requirements.

Lipton points out that people living just above this double-80
standard may be to some extent undernourished, and probably
experience hunger quite frequently. He calls them 'moderately
poor' on the grounds that the risk of physiological impairment
they face is likely to be much less than for the 'ultra-poor'. He
further estimates that 'the ultra-poor... form 10–20 per cent of
populations' in most low-income countries, and for India finds a
startling contrast between urban and rural populations. Calculat-
ing on the basis of monthly expenditure per person (MEP), he
comments that in 1972–3: '41% of India's rural households – but
under 2% of urban – fell into MEP groups averaging food/outlay
ratios above 80%' (Lipton, 1982, p.45).

In urban areas, more money is probably needed for non-food
items such as fuel, but this does not fully account for the
rural/urban difference.

Social valuations

Discussion of poverty, even more than of undernutrition, brings us back to the question of what is acceptable or otherwise to a particular nation or social group. Among several ways in which this question might be tackled, one is for the investigator himself to lay down minimum expenditures on food, clothing, fuel, housing and so on for families of different size, and to consider that those with incomes less than this are living in poverty. This is what Rowntree (1901) did in his pioneer work on poverty in Britain. In using this method, the investigator makes his own valuation of what should be regarded as unacceptable, in the light of what he knows of social norms and physiological needs for food and warmth.

Table 4.1 summarises a wide range of estimates concerning the extent of poverty in India at three dates for which information from the National Sample Survey (NSS) enables such calculations to be made. The estimates differ considerably, and have been the subject of great and continuing controversy. However, it is important to note that they are not all attempting to measure the same thing. Sukhatme (1981a,b) deals specifically with malnutrition; but Rao (1981), Dandekar (1981) and others include undernutrition within their definitions of poverty.

The table also illustrates some of the many different energy requirements figures that have been used in arriving at poverty lines. These figures are for a standard 'consumer unit', that is, a moderately active 'reference man' weighing 55 kg. Family food needs are estimated from this by counting women and children as fractional consumer units at various levels.

A rather different way of establishing criteria for the estimation of poverty is to observe how the poor express their own valuations through their behaviour when purchasing food. Boyd-Orr used this approach in his surveys of food, health and income in the UK during the 1930s (Boyd-Orr, 1937). Lipton's double-80 criterion is based on the empirical observation that in several countries, including India, almost no group of poor people allocates significantly more than 80 per cent of household expenditure to food. The 80 per cent level seems to represent a

Table 4.1 *Estimates of the extent of poverty in India based on National Sample Survey data on consumer expenditure (compare Kumar 1973)*

Authors and dates of NSS figures used	Minimum energy intake used in calculating poverty lines based on income		Cut-off level adopted as the poverty line, or to define under-nutrition	Percentage of population below the cut-off level defined	
	MJ	kcal		Rural	Urban
Bardhan (1970a, b)			Income of		
1960–1	11.3	2700	Rs 15	38	
1967–8	11.3	2700	a	53	
Dandekar and Rath (1971); Dandekar (1981)			Income of		
1960–1	9.4	2250	Rs 15 (rural)	40	
			Rs 22.5 (urban)		50
1967–8	9.4	2250	a	40	50
1971–2	9.6	2300	a	46.5[d]	
Ojha (1970)			Income of		
1960–1	9.4[c]	2250[c]	Rs 18–21	52	
1967–8	9.4[c]	2250[c]	a	70	
Rao (1981)			Income of		
1971–2	9.6[c]	2300[c]	Rs 21-24	29[b]	
Sukhatme (1981a,b)			Food intake		
1960–1			of 8.8 MJ		25–33[bd]
			Food intake		
1971–2			of 9.6 MJ	20[b]	25[b]
FAO (1977)			Food intake		
1971–2			= 1.2 × BMR	17[b]	21[b]
Lipton (1982)			80% of spending		
1972–3			on food	41	2
			Breakdown of		
1972–3			Engels's law	10–30	5–20

Notes:
a denotes that the same poverty line was used as for 1960–1, but with adjustment for inflation;   b refers to percentage below stated energy intake, not below the income poverty line;   c based on average intake;   d refers to rural and urban populations.

critical condition below which people behave as if they have no real options left: they cannot easily economise further on non-food items, nor can they manage with less food. If their income per caput falls further, forcing more cuts in spending, food and non-food items are reduced in the same proportion.

Another way of looking at this is in terms of Engel's law. When comparison is made between better-off and worse-off groups as judged by income per family member, it is found that a progressively larger percentage of family expenditure is used to buy food as one goes down the income scale. The relationship is stated by Engel's law to be a linear one, as Figure 4.3 illustrates for a particular instance. The graph also shows that below the point where 80 per cent of spending is devoted to food, actual expenditures diverge from the sloping line, and the law ceases to be obeyed. Indeed, the point where Engel's law ceases to be applicable might itself be used to define an 'ultra-poverty' line (V.B. Rao, 1981), although this cannot be done with much precision. Using the NSS data for India, Lipton (1982, p.45) concluded that 'for the poorest 10–30 per cent in rural areas and 5–20 per cent in towns, Engel's law does not apply'.

The larger proportion of rural people identified by Lipton as living in ultra-poverty is again significant, especially in view of the higher mortality rates (including infant mortality) recorded in rural areas. Yet according to HCS data, rural food intakes are much the same as urban populations. Noting this, Lipton suggests that for rural people, food energy requirements are greater. There is more heavy work to be done, not only in agriculture but in carrying water and other tasks, and there are more pregnancies. As we observed in Chapter 1, malnutrition occurs at different levels of intake in different environments. By contrast, if a single, fixed food energy requirement is assumed for everybody, poverty and undernutrition seem more prevalent in *urban* India.

It will be apparent that two sorts of data are used in these various attempts to define criteria for the nutritional aspect of poverty: observations of people's behaviour, and conclusions drawn from scientific models of energy needs. The way these data are combined depends on a variety of assumptions and

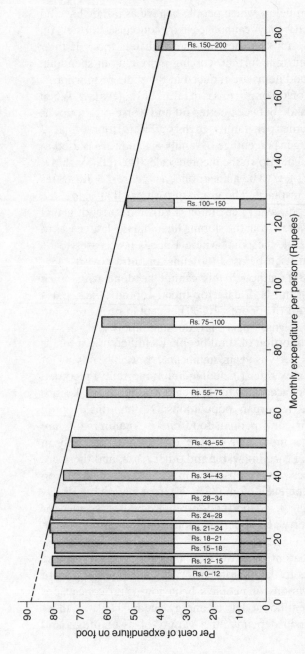

Figure 4.3   Monthly consumer expenditure per person (MEP) in *rural* areas of Maharashtra, October 1972–September 1973

Notes: Each vertical bar represents one MEP class. The modal class in the survey, with 1051 households, was that for Rs. 34–43 per person. There were only 74 households spending less than Rs. 13 per person, and only 25 in the Rs. 150–200 class.

Source: NSS data, twenty-seventh round 1972–3, *Sarvekshana*, January 1979, quoted by Lipton 1982, table 6.

valuations. Conventional nutritional requirement figures, based on observing healthy populations whose intakes are not constrained by poverty, provide one type of behavioural evidence. These data are then frequently used in conjunction with some form of 'genetic potential' model, and in relation to Table 4.1, lead to the estimates which place 50 per cent and more of the Indian population below various poverty lines.

By contrast, Sukhatme (1981a,b) uses a version of the individual adaptability model, with minimum intake fixed and no allowance made for differences in adaptation between rural and urban groups and sub-groups. The proportion of the population below the poverty line is then given as between 20 per cent and 25 per cent (Table 4.1). The same approach was used by FAO (1977): a critical limit of response or adaptation, estimated at 1.2 × BMR (see Chapter 3 above). The authors themselves applied this level to the 1971–2 data from India and estimated that around 17 per cent of rural people should be regarded as suffering from undernutrition at this level. The estimate is very close to Sukhatme's figure.

Lipton (1982) relies much more than the other authors on observed behaviour that is symptomatic of critically low levels of food intake, and by implication gives less weight to any of the scientific models. Assuming that the real extent of adaptability in individuals is reflected in their behaviour, Lipton's results may well come closest to reflecting real limits of adaptability or response in the populations he considers. This makes his conclusion about rural/urban differentials doubly important.

Observing people's food purchasing behaviour falls a long way short of the 'dialogue' between scientists, planners, and consumers of food we earlier envisaged (p.77). But taking account of behavioural evidence is an important way of at least beginning an exploration of social valuations regarding food needs; it points to some of the more extreme limits of what is acceptable in a given society.

Problems of cut-off points: *a* poverty lines

Amartya Sen (1974) has commented that the poor of India 'may not be accustomed to receiving much help', but they are 'beginning to get used to being counted'. Knowing that precisely X per cent of India's or the world's population falls below a certain poverty line does not necessarily help alleviate that poverty. Thus the number of 'ultra-poor' people identified by Lipton matters less than the way he is also able to point out concentrations of rural poverty in certain places – on inferior land in Bihar, Assam, Orissa and West Bengal, for example, or among the low-caste and tribal landless in western India. These latter are the kind of facts on which some sort of action might be based. We shall take up these ideas again later.

Scott and Mathew (1983) suggest in a study of poverty in Kerala that the variables relating to poverty, 'should be express-ed initially in terms of a distribution', without reference to any particular poverty line, because the choice of a cut-off point is always relative to the socio-economic context. They go on to argue that, 'it may be more helpful to administrators or local village committees whose job it is to provide relief or ameliorate conditions, to decide on their own critical points ... in the light of ... resources and needs, and with full knowledge, rather than the half knowledge provided by a poverty line'.

This is an approach to be commended wherever it can be adopted, because once cut-off points have been defined and found to be useful, they are often taken over and used out of context by other investigators. Poverty lines based on income, for instance, are not necessarily accurate indicators of nutritional risk. Rigidity in the use of an indicator implies that no dialogue is taking place about what cut-off points might best represent 'unacceptable' conditions. Furthermore, in a country in which development policies are achieving at least some of their goals, we would expect the borderline between acceptable and un-acceptable risk to be raised continuously. Poverty lines should then be adjusted from year to year. Actually the poverty line used by the Indian Planning Commission is based on 1961–2 real prices. And another example of what ought *not* to happen is provided by Woolf (1946) and Walker and Church (1978): Rowntree's 'absolute minimum for survival' poverty line con-tinued to be used in Britain for a period of over forty years and indeed is still the basis of state social security and welfare intervention. One danger with Lipton's double-80 criterion is that its evident usefulness and apparent objectivity may give it a similar permanence.

Problems of cut off points: *b* anthropometry

Similar considerations apply to the cut-off points used in connection with anthropometric data. Gomez *et al*. (1956) used hospital mortality results to define a cut-off point at 60 per cent of standard weight-for-age, and described children below this level as suffering from 'severe' or 'third degree' malnutrition. This cut-off point and these terms have been used by many subsequent authors, and have become part of the vocabulary of nutrition; they are summarised in Table 4.2 along with similar classifications used with other anthropometric indicators.

The use of Harvard standards for heights and weights was mentioned in Chapter 2. The standards were originally derived from measurements of several thousand American children, and are presented as sets of age-standardised centiles. These should be regarded as probability statements. The 90th centile for any measurement is a set of numerical values below which we would expect to find 90 per cent of a sample, with only 10 per cent above. It thus represents a condition well above average, and in a set of data representing body weights, the 90th centile would correspond to about 115 per cent of standard weight-for-age.

At the other end of the scale, the 1st centile might be used as a cut-off point in weight-for-age to identify children who are at risk in some way. There is a probability of only 0.01 that a healthy individual would have this weight, so if we found that *all* the individuals in a sample were on or below the 1st centile, we would have good reason to think that not all of them were 'well nourished'. In the Harvard distribution, body weights of individuals in the 1st centile are near 60 per cent of those of individuals in the 50th centile – that is, they are about 60 per cent of 'standard'. And as we have said, 60 per cent weight-for-age is very widely taken as the cut-off point identifying individuals who

Table 4.2   *Panel showing examples of Harvard Standards for anthropometric data and illustrating some classifications commonly used.*

Weight-for-age

(a)   Harvard 50th centile weights for young children of both sexes at representative ages.

Age/years	0	0.5	1	2	3	4	5
Weight/kg	3.4	7.4	9.9	12.4	14.5	16.5	18.4

(b)   Interpretation of weights below Harvard Standard 50th centile

Weight as % of Harvard standard	Gomez classification	
> 90	normal	{ includes individuals in the 25th centile and above
75 – 90	{ mild undernutrition (1st degree)	
60 – 75	{ moderate undernutrition (2nd degree)	
<60	severe (3rd degree)	{ includes only individuals in the 1st centile

---

have a low probability of being 'healthy', and therefore a high probability of 'severe malnutrition' (Table 4.2).

These cut-off points are given because they are so widely used, but we also need to recall that their significance is always relative to our circumstances, resources and purpose (Chapter 2). In screening a particular population, for example, we might have resources to treat all those on the 10th centile and below. This means that we would use 85 per cent weight-for-age as a cut-off, regardless of how it relates to the Gomez classification.

It is sometimes possible to attach greater significance to a cut-off point if it defines conditions where some particular risk begins to increase steeply. For example, in the group of children studied by Chen *et al.* (1980) in Bangladesh mentioned in Chapter 2, the numbers of deaths occurring in the two years after anthropometric data were recorded has the distribution relative

Height-for-age

Harvard 50th centile heights or lengths for young children of both sexes at representative ages.

Age/years	0	0.5	1	2	3	4	5
Length/cm	50.4	65.8	74.7	87.1	96.0	103.3	109.0

Weight-for-height

The Waterlow classification (Waterlow 1972, 1976) combines two indicators, weight-for-height, and height-for-age. Children of low weight-for-height are referred to as 'wasted'; those of low height-for-age are termed 'stunted'.

	Weight-for-height	
	More than 80% Harvard Standard	Less than 80% Harvard Standard
Height-for-age		
More than 90% Harvard Standard	classed as NORMAL	classed as WASTED
Less than 90% Harvard Standard	classed as STUNTED	highest risk category: STUNTED AND WASTED

to weight-for-age which is shown in Figure 4.4. There is an 'elbow' in the curve where mortality risk begins to rise rapidly, and this break in the curve is located at values of weight-for-age around 60–65 per cent of Harvard standard. Bairagi (1982) quotes similar data from a group of Indian children studied by Kielman and McCord (1978), and discusses statistical considerations to locate the 'best cut-off point' more precisely on the elbow of the curve. As Figure 4.4 shows, the point is not the same for the two communities. Moreover, the Narangwal study also showed that the shape of the curve depended on the age of children measured: risk of death for a given nutritional status decreased with age. The possibilities of using anthropometric measurements as indicators and the statistical, rather than value issues involved are discussed further by Habicht *et al.* (1982), and

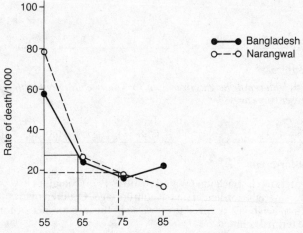

Figure 4.4   Variation of death rate vs weight-for-age for two groups of children: Bangladesh (children aged 12–24 months), Narangwal, India (children aged 0–36 months)
Notes: The vertical lines at 63 and 73 per cent weight-for-age represent Bairagi's view of the 'best cut-off points' for nutritional monitoring.
Sources: Bangladesh, Chen *et al*. 1980; Narangwal, Kielmann and McCord 1978; diagram after Bairagi 1982.

also by Trowbridge and Staehling (1980) and Eusebio and Nube (1981).

Another question that arises is whether standards derived in one country can be used to evaluate individuals in another. Some studies indicate that there are small differences in growth pattern between Africans, Asians and Caucasians, although these only appear after 5 years of age (e.g. Hiernaux, 1964; Jelliffe, 1966; Habicht *et al*., 1974). We may ask whether, even if all human groups have basically the same genetic growth potential, national standards should not still be used because they take account of environmental and economic differences.

Much discussion has been given to these questions, but to answer them we need to come back to a basic point. The actual value of weight-for-age at which children's mortality rates increase sharply can be called X kg. On the Harvard standard, X is 60 per cent weight-for-age. Any standards could be used to define 'malnutrition'; cut-off points may be chosen according to measured risks, or to resources available for allocating treatments, or to suit some other purpose. If such procedures are consistently followed, it does not matter very much what standard values are used, as long as they are derived from a large sample, with acceptable methods of measurement.

In any case, as we saw in Chapter 2, there is no unambiguous way of fixing points on the scale so that 'high risk' are sharply divided from 'normal' individuals. For any fixed point, there will be some healthy individuals who fall below it, so in a practical situation where action is contemplated, there will be some healthy people who are treated as if they are sick, or at risk of death.

Although it makes sense to use the 'elbow' of the risk curve as a cut-off point, we should adopt this procedure with caution, for two reasons. Firstly, to apply a statistical test in order to establish the best cut-off point may pre-empt the dialogue we have mentioned as necessary in making social valuations. Risks are not zero for children who are better than 60–65 per cent weight-for-age, and we cannot be sure that the 'elbow' of the curve coincides with the view of these risks taken either by planners, or by parents of the children concerned. It is also often the case, however, that those whose children fall into the extreme, worst category are excluded from any intervention or any dialogue at all. Where there is an option of spending more money in order to provide treatments (or food) for extra children, those who provide the funds might also have a view – they might wish the treatments to be given even though the children who benefit are in low-risk category.

Secondly, we should note that a cut-off point defined by reference to mortality risk in one part of the world may not be applicable to morbidity risks in the same population groups, nor applicable at all in any useful way to children in a different region or continent (Kasongo Project Team, 1983). Investigating the incidence and prevalence of diarrhoea among children in Nigeria, Tomkins (1981) found that the *frequency* of diarrhoea was no greater for children of low weight-for-age than for others, but that such children took significantly longer to recover from each attack. Weight-for-height proved to be more effective as an indicator of the risk of an attack. Among children who were below 80 per cent standard weight-for-height, episodes of diarrhoea were 1.47 times more likely than among those above this level. Chen *et al.* (1981c) found similar results. Reddy *et al.* (1976), and Cunningham-Rundles (1982) among others, have looked at the association between resistance to infection and nutritional status.

In these circumstances there are no clear-cut answers about which indicator to use, and with what cut-off points. Parents might be worried about the high incidence of some particular illness, while educationists point out that slow recovery from another disease is holding back children's learning. Different indicators and fixed points would be needed to respond to these different concerns. Once again, therefore, several points of view must be considered before social valuations of risk can be fully appreciated. And as in other instances we have considered, the deciding factors about cut-off points must include dialogue concerning the relative importance of risks of different aspects of malnutrition, and a clear idea about the purpose for which the indicator is being used and the resources available.

PART TWO

The Causes of
Malnutrition

'It... places the emphasis on *man*, and endeavours to
study him in, and in relation to, his environment ...
economic, nutritional, occupational.'

John A. Ryle, on epidemiology as an aspect of 'social medicine'
(see Ryle, 1948, p.11)

5 Multiple causes in malnutrition*

A focus on people

The direction in which previous chapters have pointed is towards the need for a comparative understanding of malnutrition as it occurs in different sectors of society, and as it is affected by geographic, environmental and disease factors. We approached this conclusion by a negative route, noting the limitations of more conventional approaches. Measurements of average food consumption do not tell us about social patterns of underconsumption; requirements figures do not in practice tell us about which food intakes are likely to lead to malnutrition. Taking a more constructive approach, we may now say that our goal in studying the social distribution of malnutrition is to understand how people become malnourished in terms of processes within society. We may then hope to find out who these people are and what policies or changes in society might help them (Joy and Payne, 1975; Payne, 1982).

Two major themes in any such study must be the *distribution* of malnutrition in the population, discussed below in Chapter 6, and *causality*, dealt with here. An example of limited but pioneer

---

*This chapter is based on material prepared by Peter Cutler, David Nabarro and Philip Payne; see especially Cutler (1982b) and Nabarro (1982). We are also indebted to a teaching text on epidemiology by Jones *et al.* (1982) for one way of presenting the concept of multiple causes.

work on both aspects was carried out in the UK in the 1930s, under the banner of 'social medicine'. In one study, begun in 1932, James Spence studied malnutrition among children in the northern British city of Newcastle-upon-Tyne. His work 'amongst the poorest classes' led him to think that three factors were interacting: infectious disease, the effects of poor housing, and inadequate diet. He described the symptoms he saw in the children as 'apparent malnutrition' to express his view that inadequate food was not always the prime cause (Spence, 1960).

The relative importance of infection, environment and food in causing the problems with which we are concerned has been a continuing subject for debate. For example, Gopalan (1983) accepts that environmental factors often influence the growth of children in ways that lead to malnutrition, but argues that: 'There is no way by which environment can influence growth and development except by conditioning and modifying the availability of essential nutrients... at the cellular level.' Thus retarded growth: 'is a reflection of *under-nutrition* and of *nothing else*' (Gopalan's italics). However, poor housing can have an effect by inducing 'stress situations, like exposure to cold or infections which condition the net availability of nutrients at the cellular level'.

In his work among children in Newcastle, Spence recognised the same issue. The aim should be to study, 'how disease and social circumstances are related', and to work at a level that 'places the emphasis on *man*, and endeavours to study him in, and in relation to his environment ... economic, nutritional, occupational' (Spence, 1960; quoting Ryle, 1948).

Our argument is that we chiefly require better understanding of these factors at a level accessible to policy interventions such as improvements in housing or more ample food supplies. Indeed, we might need to know which of these options is likely to give more benefit to a particular social group, and at what cost.

This is not an easy set of issues to pursue, however. The environmental circumstances of people's lives are very varied, and a causal analysis of nutritional problems could rapidly become an excessively cumbersome analysis of the human condition (Payne, 1976). One strategy adopted in the past to avoid such complexities was to identify those few symptoms or combinations of symptoms for which simple nutritional explanations do seem to work. During the period from 1930 to 1950, nutritionists following this procedure were successful in identifying several vitamin deficiencies, such as pellagra (niacin deficiency) among impoverished people living mainly on maize in the United States. They also identified thiamin deficiency among polished-rice eaters in Japan, and inadequate vitamin A in the diets of low-income groups in Newfoundland. These investigations were all followed by fortification projects, and over subsequent years, deficiency symptoms in the populations declined. A careful historical analysis shows that in all these situations, however, the decline was as much associated with rapid social and economic improvements as it was with the nutritional intervention: indeed in all cases the decline was already well under way before the programmes were started. However, these interventions established a pattern for public health nutrition in the 1950s, and it was against this background of apparent success that the disease of small children called kwashiorkor gradually came to be accepted as due to protein deficiency alone. We saw in Chapter 3 that more recent research has largely disposed of this view.

Some diseases which seem explicable in terms of nutrient deficiencies are distressingly widespread. The documentation for India's sixth five-year plan quotes lack of vitamin A in diets as the cause of widespread xerophthalmia, leading to blindness in the most severe cases (Government of India, 1981). Nutritional anaemia and goitre are often cited as the two other most prevalent deficiency diseases affecting the poor in many developing countries (FAO, 1977).

Nothing that is said in this book should be taken as minimising the significance of these forms of malnutrition. Our argument is simply that the model of single dietary deficiency causes used to understand them is of limited application. It is based on an epidemiological approach, certainly, but one which lacks adequate means of analysing the multiple causes of disease. For example, according to FAO (1977), nutritional anaemia affects at least 20 per cent of children in developing countries and even more adult women; among men the prevalence could be around 10 per cent. This does not necessarily mean their diets are deficient in iron however. One study of labourers employed on road works in north India, for example, found that although there was no correlation between work output and energy intake, reduced levels of output observed for some labourers were significantly correlated with anaemia (Tandon *et al.*, 1975). Surprisingly, perhaps, the diet eaten by these men included 'generous' helpings of lentils, and supplied more than three times the recommended daily allowance of iron. As with many other people eating largely vegetarian diets, the problem seemed to be one of malabsorption of iron rather than inadequate intake. In many social groups there is also a heavy burden of parasitic disease due mainly to poor sanitation, and this gives rise to iron loss. Thus even a superficial account of one type of anaemia leads us to notice other causes apart from deficient food intakes. (For example, see M.C. Latham *et al.*, 1983.)

With other illnesses that are conventionally attributed to poor nutrition, causal explanations become even more complex. Referring again to kwashiorkor in young children, it is becoming increasingly clear that this is not a problem of low food intake alone (Whitehead, 1977; Lunn *et al.*, 1979; Martorell *et al.*, 1980). Modern research has come to focus on diarrhoeal infections as a precipitating factor, and there is a danger that those who think in terms of single causes will now rather easily fall into the habit of speaking about infection as 'the cause' of malnutrition. However, the precise mechanisms by which diarrhoea leads to this type of malnutrition are uncertain. Also while some investigators (Rutishauser, 1974; Mata *et al.*, 1977; Tomkins 1983) suggest that anorexia is the main cause, others stress that, during diarrhoea, there is malabsorption of nutrients due to abnormality in gut flora and function (Gracey *et al.*, 1977; Rowland, 1981); yet others (Tomkins *et al.*, 1983) have shown that the fever associated with infections raises the body's requirement for dietary energy.

In examining the nutritional problems of young children, we first have to remember that their energy needs are proportionately higher than those of adults. When children are breast-fed, mothers produce adequate amounts of milk to support growth in the first weeks after birth. However, low energy supply may begin to affect growth in some children from as early as three months. In many developing countries, children who are solely breast-fed gain weight more slowly than expected when compared with more privileged populations (Waterlow *et al.*, 1980). The seasonal variability in mothers' dietary intake in a West African rural community has also been shown to influence milk output (Paul *et al.*, 1979; Rowland *et al.*, 1981; Prentice *et al.*, 1981; Roberts *et al.*, 1982). Whatever the circumstances, most mothers are unable to produce sufficient milk to sustain adequate child growth after six months, so by then supplementation with other foods should have begun.

The period when childrens' health is most in danger starts at three months and lasts until they can feed themselves, perhaps when about three years old (Khan, 1984). During this period, there are several feeding practices which can have an influence on child nutrition. One is the age at which food supplements (specifically non-milk supplements) are introduced into the child's diet. Another is the method of preparation. Foods prepared in the home – whether supplied by a commercial company in a tin or prepared using village technology – frequently become contaminated with bacteria from the water supply or the domestic environment.

In some places where weaning foods are mostly cereal gruels, local fuel shortages (and sometimes pressure on the mothers' time) make it impossible to cook frequent meals for small children. Larger batches of food are therefore prepared in advance and kept for long periods, during which the bacteria multiply. Thus the foods used in the earliest stages of weaning have sometimes been found to have higher levels of contamination than food eaten by other members of the family (Rowland *et al.*, 1978). The result is often diarrhoea, and children aged less than six months are especially vulnerable. For them, diarrhoea can lead very quickly to dehydration, and death may follow soon after.

When weaning begins, the food must be liquid. This often means that it is mixed with large volumes of water, and its energy density, as a result, is very low. If the child is ill and appetite falls, intake will also be low. Mothers who cannot use energy-dense foods (such as fats, oils and even sugars) will have difficulty in maintaining their children's energy intake. Weight lost during the illness will not easily be regained unless the child is given considerably more than the normal maintenance energy requirements.

In all circumstances, but especially during illness, small children need to be fed frequently during the day – and frequent feeds are particularly important when bulky or watery foods are used. Mothers may have difficulty in doing this if they are working in the fields, or when they have other children to look after. Thus limited time available to mothers may be an important constraint on children's food intake.

Simply by reviewing these problems which mothers in poor social groups commonly encounter in feeding their infants, we can form a picture of the many factors that may influence a child's health and nutritional status. If the child falls ill, it is meaningless to argue about whether low food intake or infection plays the larger part; moreover, it is also clear that other contributory causes may include environmental conditions (fuel supply, sanitation), and social and emotional pressures arising from the mother's work load. A diagram such as Figure 5.1 summarises these conclusions in a way which makes it difficult to revert to single-cause thinking. The diagram also helps to indicate the policy options available to those who wish to ameliorate matters. For example, it shows that providing the mother with better baby foods or teaching her about hygiene will only deal with a small part of the overall problem, and not necessarily the most critical one. The extra food or education may be of little help if the mother still has insufficient time to prepare foods properly, or lacks fuel to cook them. Thus, as we emphasised earlier in the chapter, it is important in any given circumstance to understand as closely as possible the limiting factors, open to intervention, which affect a child's well-being.

Illness in an agrarian environment

These points can be put into context by reference to studies in

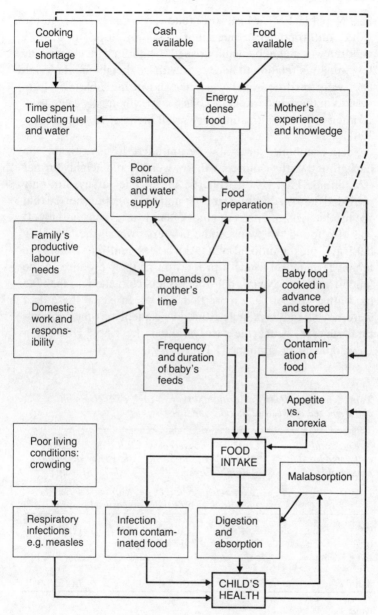

Figure 5.1 Summary of factors affecting the nutrition of small children

east Nepal in 1975, which were followed up in 1977–81. In this work, anthropometric measurements were used to identify children who might be malnourished. Children with abnormally low weight in relation to height, or with low height in relation to age, were recorded in the manner shown in Table 5.1. Individuals in these two categories of slow growth mostly came from farming families cultivating very small areas of land (Nabarro, 1981).

Socio-economic surveys were initiated to investigate the background of the children with low weights and heights further (Conlin and Falk, 1979; Roberts, 1981). The surveys not only provided data on different sizes of land holding, but showed that the productivity of different kinds of land varies substantially. It was also found that while some farmers own all the land they cultivate, plus additional plots which they rent out, others are tenant farmers returning a proportion of their produce to the landlord as rent. Nearly half the farmers cultivate less than 0.5 ha; only a quarter have more than 1.0 ha. In Nepal these data were not already available from government or other agricultural surveys, hence the surveys under the Khosi Hills Area Development Programme (KHARDEP).

Table 5.1   *KHARDEP Nutrition Survey, Nepal, 1979 (Data on children aged between 12 months and 5 years.)*

Area of land cultivated by the household	Children who were less than 80% of standard weight-for-height[1]		Children who were less than 85% of standard height-for-age[1]	
	Number measured	*Number affected*	*Number measured*	*Number affected*
0.0 – 0.5 ha	55	9 (16%)	54	17 (32%)
0.51 – 1.0 ha	98	12 (12%)	96	28 (30%)
over 1.0 ha	168	3 (2%)	152	31 (20%)
Total	321	24 (7%)	302	76 (25%)

Note:
[1]Standard weights and heights were derived from WHO/NAS tables; see WHO (1979).

In Nepal, the majority of the rain falls during the summer months (May to September). The maize harvest starts in July; the rice harvest on farms with irrigated lands is complete by late November or early December. Many farmers normally produce only about half of their household grain requirements on their own land and therefore need to obtain grain from other sources between February and July. Some farmers earn money to buy food by taking casual work on the larger holdings, or by doing building work, portering (carrying goods into the hills), or occasionally by blacksmithing, tailoring and so on. They may sell animals or animal products, and when food shortages are severe, they take loans. The result is that during food shortage months, small farmers' households are likely to experience a fall in consumption of animal products and perhaps staple foods also. In addition, *all* the adults and older children will usually be fully committed to income-earning activities; some may go away in search of work. Some families have to sell their assets bit by bit, slowly getting poorer and further into debt. The farmers with the smallest amounts of land experience substantial deficits each year, and are often disinvesting by selling animals and mortgaging land.

An additional problem for nearly everybody is that with each generation, land available to the household decreases. It is divided equally among the sons and there is little new land coming into cultivation.

In 1977, the Nepal Children's Organisation established a small child care programme in the centre of the Kosi Hills area where the socio-economic surveys were undertaken. Within the first year of operation, it became clear that there was pronounced seasonal variation in children's attendance at the clinic in Dhankuta (Nepal Children's Organisation, 1980). The highest attendances occurred during the summer months (up to July). Case histories of child attenders who were markedly below expected weight revealed that a high proportion (but by no means all) came from families who experienced substantial food deficits. Their condition was frequently accompanied by infection, or a family crisis (like the death of a parent), or the birth of a new child. Thus a multiplicity of causes was clearly evident.

A community health programme was initiated in the village in which detailed family profiles were recorded (McLean, 1981). All homes were visited regularly, and over 95 per cent of the children in the village were seen at least once a year and often much more. Monthly 'prevalence' figures were calculated and field workers weighed and measured children. In these ways, a fairly comprehensive set of epidemiological data was collected during 1978–9, leading to the following general conclusions:

1. Child weight-gains were greatest between July and December; some 79 per cent of total annual weight gain occurred then.
2. Diarrhoea was frequently encountered in May, June and July; in 1979 there was also a measles outbreak during February, March and April.
3. The prevalence of conjunctival xerosis (a sign of vitamin A deficiency) was highest in May–July (Padfield and Nabarro, 1981).
4. The number of children below 80 per cent of expected weight-for-height was highest in August and September, falling to zero in November/December and rising between February and June.

It seems from these studies, therefore, that diarrhoeal disease in children accompanies the first of the summer rains; and that child weight-gain is maximal after the maize harvest (this village grows little rice). Nutritional problems in children either coincide with or come shortly after the period of maximum food shortage, which is also the time when diarrhoea incidence is highest. Thus the effects of low food intake and infection are compounded.

Other studies in nearby villages (Devkota, 1981; Rickelton, 1981) have confirmed that in the early monsoon months, adults are particularly likely to be hard at work in their fields or labouring for cash. Men and women are all very busy and time available for domestic activities is constrained. Thus child malnutrition in these villages is likely to be encountered during the months when women are working hardest, infection is commonest, and food is in particularly short supply. At this time, too, market prices for some foods – particularly grain and clarified butter – also tend to be highest and communications are hampered by the rains. So again the picture is one of several contributory causes or risk factors interacting, each exacerbating the influence of the others. It is difficult to disentangle the results and say that either food shortage, or diarrhoea, or constraints on mothers' time is most crucial. Many others who have done detailed studies on malnutrition in a particular community would come to the same conclusions.

What is needed is a systematic procedure for identifying the various contributory causes of malnutrition and of comprehending the nature of their interactions. There are in fact various different ways of approaching the problems of causal analysis, and in what follows we shall describe some of them, but not with the objective of identifying the best methodology. In any practical situation it is likely that a number of different techniques in combination will be found useful. The objective is to devise a model, or conceptual framework which will enable us to ask more effective questions about how people become malnourished, and how these processes may be modified by interventions. Perhaps the most important point to make at this stage, however, is that none of these procedures should be seen as devices for identifying *the ultimate cause* of malnutrition.

Modelling multiple causes

The work on malnutrition in Nepal emphasised the distribution of the problem among the different types of cultivator and across the seasons, and we shall refer to this aspect further in the next chapter. We might pursue further the question of the contributory causes of malnutrition in either of two ways.

Firstly, we might extend the descriptive process by using a diagrammatic method such as that illustrated by Figure 5.1. Secondly, we might resort to statistical techniques of the kind that are widely used in other branches of epidemiology (Jones *et al.*, 1982), or more generally in dealing with social statistics (Blalock, 1979).

The study of mortality among children in Bangladesh (Chen *et al.*, 1980) which was cited in Chapters 2 and 4 provides us with some data which becomes more comprehensible when viewed within the context of Figure 5.1. Among 112 children who died during the two-year period covered by the work, the illness which preceded death was recorded as diarrhoea in 41 instances, measles in 19, and 'other infections' in 20. For part of their analysis, Chen and his colleagues divided the children into 'better nourished' and 'malnourished' groups, using 65 per cent of standard weight-for-age as the criterion separating the two. The overall death rate was much greater in the malnourished group, and in particular, the death rate associated with diarrhoea was 3.7 times greater. In a subsequent review, Chen *et al.* (1981a) took this as evidence that many of the deaths attributed to diarrhoea and other infections ought to be regarded as caused by malnutrition. They added that most deaths due to malnutrition in other, similar circumstances, 'are likely to be attributed to infections, among which diarrhoea and measles are most prominent'.

This conclusion, however, appears to disregard evidence from the same research that children in the 'malnourished' group were more likely to die when they were also living in crowded housing. If this were to be stressed, one might well argue that many deaths attributed to diarrhoea and measles ought to be regarded as due to housing conditions. Chen *et al.* classed a house as 'crowded' if the family occupied less than 22.5 m^2 (or 242 ft^2); it may often be that where there is less floor space, children are more exposed to respiratory infections and hygiene is less good. A higher incidence of measles and diarrhoea is thus to be expected.

It would make sense to regard crowded housing and poor nutritional status as two of several 'risk factors' tending to increase the likelihood of death, but there is little point in manipulating statistics to 'prove' that one or other is more important. As Joy (1981) comments, investigation of 'causes' is often sterile if one loses sight of the system within which the malnutrition is being generated. Weight-for-age below the 65 per cent level and crowding may both be useful indicators of the state of this system at a single point in time, but are best seen as representing underlying processes rather than as independent causes of illness or death of the sort which many discussions seek to identify.

Analysis of processes within the household needs to be extended by comparisons between different kinds of household. The well-known survey of a rural population in the Punjab described by Levinson (1974) dealt with a society in which the occurrence of various environmental, occupational and nutritional risk factors was rather different. When comparison was made between landless families and children from households owning some land, it was found that proportionately three times as many children in the landless group were below 60 per cent of standard weight-for-age. In commenting on the results, FAO (1977) stressed that low weight-for-age correlated much more strongly with the incidence of infection than with diet. Among the population covered by the survey, there were not only farmers and labourers, but also people with 'service jobs'. Seasonal fluctuations in work load could be very different for these occupational groups, leading to difference in the pressures on mothers' time and consequent variations in the feeding of young children.

This kind of analysis, which stresses the importance of socio-economic differences between households, is complementary to an understanding of the causal processes operating within the household. Its importance is that it further extends our ability to distinguish the likely impact on malnutrition of policies or interventions which affect different classes or categories of household. In Chapter 6 these ideas will be developed further in a discussion about how to devise 'functional classifications' of households.

If a statistical analysis is thought desirable, then it must clearly be one that is capable of accommodating several variables (Blalock, 1979). An example is the use of correlation analysis in the study of north Indian road workers previously quoted (Tandon *et al.*, 1975). The physical work output of 198 individuals was measured while they carried out a task which involved digging and carrying sand. Height, weight and arm circumference were measured for each individual. Fasting blood samples were taken, and a number of biochemical parameters were measured. Records of food intake were also kept.

A first step in analysing the results was to calculate correlation coefficients for all the variables, setting out the results in a matrix (Table 5.2). Correlations close enough to be significant at the 5 per cent level were then identified. For example, work output was significantly but weakly correlated with body weight, indicating that the larger individuals tended to do more work than the smaller and thinner men.

For one group of road workers, recruited locally in northern Uttar Pradesh, there was a significant correlation between work output and red blood cell iron measured by hematocrit values. As mentioned earlier, this suggests that anaemia had an effect on the work done. However, no similar effect was apparent in a second group of workers, so the correlation for both groups combined was small. The major limitation of correlation analysis as a means of modelling multiple causes is that a significant correlation shows that two variables are *associated*, but does not prove that one *causes* the other. If two quantities are increasing with the passage of time, they will always be positively correlated, often strongly, even when they are entirely unrelated. Thus we may sometimes learn more from the lack of a correlation. Referring again to the road workers, we may observe that there was no correlation between food energy intake and work output (Table 5.2). As Tandon comments, this provides, 'a further rebuttal of some long held concepts'.

There are other reasons why this type of exercise is only of

Table 5.2 *Part of the matrix prepared by Tandon et al. (1975) to show correlations between the work output of 198 labourers and the variables shown* (Correlation coefficients underlined are significant at the 5 per cent level.)

Variable	Work output	Hemato-crit	Height	Body weight	Serum iron	Energy intake
Work output	1.000					
Hematocrit	0.024	1.000				
Height	0.087	0.082	1.000			
Body weight	0.275	−0.006	0.585	1.000		
Serum iron	0.009	0.138	−0.040	−0.062	1.000	
Energy intake	−0.047	0.128	0.114	0.027	−0.093	1.000

limited value in the study of food-related illness, however. In planning interventions that will help prevent such illness, what matters is often the *relationship* of the causal influences rather than their magnitudes. There are many different kinds of interaction by which one contributory cause may modify, deflect, or alternatively, reinforce other causal influences, and what is required is the concept of a network of relationships between different influences, not simply the measurement of correlations between them. This network concept is sometimes difficult to deal with verbally. When that is the case, a diagrammatic approach to multiple-cause modelling such as that presented in Figure 5.1 has obvious advantages.

Thus *simultaneity* is one type of relationship between causal factors which we need to identify. Low seasonal food intakes might have less obviously damaging effects if they occurred at times of year when diarrhoeal infections and measles were infrequent. The problem for many people is that the impact of seasonality is to make these factors coincide.

When we come to consider Figure 5.2, we shall also need to examine influences which partly *cancel* one another. However, factors which reinforce one another are usually of greater interest, and while the reinforcing effect may sometimes occur because of simultaneity, *feedback* is probably more commonly encountered. Figure 5.1 includes examples of feedback at the point where the child's ill-health is shown to lead to anorexia or malabsorption. Inadequate nutrition is reinforced when anorexia due to infection leads a malnourished child to refuse food.

Many other kinds of interaction between contributory causes are possible. Some factors may prove to be necessary but not sufficient as causes of a particular outcome; some may be sufficient in themselves. Some affect the *rate* at which a problem develops, whereas others *initiate* it. Some factors may serve to tip the balance in a situation between sharply contrasting outcomes, while others intensify an existing trend. Representations of the different types of causal network that result, using a variety of diagrammatic conventions, can be seen in many writings on systems theory, but the explicit development of what have been called 'problem diagrams' or 'multiple-cause diagrams' is fairly

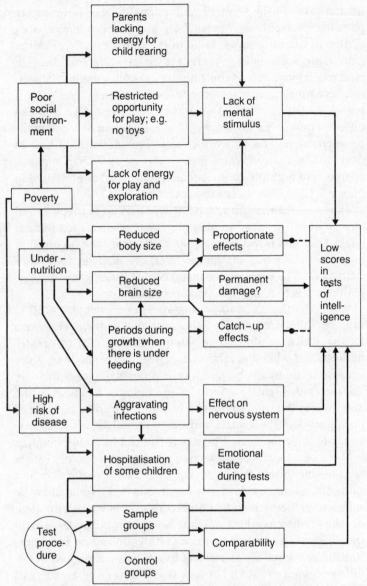

Figure 5.2   Factors affecting the observed association between under-nutrition and low scores in tests of intelligence

Notes: * denotes effects likely to cancel.

recent, and so is their application to such problems as perinatal health care or the cause of disease (Smith and Hagard, 1982; Jones *et al.*, 1982).

We may take the idea a little further by using it to analyse another assertion that is sometimes made about the effects of malnutrition, namely that the mental development of children may be retarded. Among various kinds of evidence, work on laboratory animals has shown that undernutrition at critical periods (such as the perinatal period) may have a long-term effect on brain development. On the other hand, animals that are undernourished after weaning have 'normal' brain function. In man, the vulnerable period extends from before birth and continues during the first twelve months after birth (Dobbing and Widdowson, 1965; Winick and Noble, 1966). Autopsies of children who have died after severe malnutrition show that their brains are smaller and have lower DNA content than normal children (Brown, 1965; Winnick and Rosso, 1969a,b). However, children exhibiting such physical features are usually retarded in other respects, because growth of the body has also been held back. Thus the brain although small in absolute terms may in fact be appropriately sized in proportion to the rest of the body, and a diagram such as Figure 5.2 will need to show this preservation of proportionality. We will also need to show that some infections, such as gastro-enteritis, may inhibit the development of the nervous system (Latham, 1974).

These studies do not prove that stunting of the size of the brain adversely affects intelligence. Yet, there have been other physiological and psychological studies which have shown that poor scores in intelligence tests are regularly produced by children who have been the victims of severe protein-energy malnutrition. Even if one accepts that low scores in tests indicate low 'intelligence', this does not show that malnutrition is by itself a cause of mental retardation. Cravioto and Robles (1965), for example, have drawn a general conclusion from studies in Mexico and Guatemala that the earlier malnutrition occurs in a child, the worse the retardation of intellectual development. However, it seems likely that recovery is possible over the long-term, so that there appears to be a 'catch-up' effect and the association subsequently disappears. Such a pattern of development was found by Champakan *et al.* (1968) in India.

Impacts of poverty

The above studies of children's mental development are cross-sectional, and do not establish any causal links. The children studied inevitably came from homes in which there was previous chronic poverty, so they had presumably suffered from many disadvantages in addition to, or as a result of, insufficient food. Among these we might expect to notice reduced ability of children to explore the environment (an important part of the learning process) due to energy deficits in infancy. We might further consider whether parents are able to devote time and energy to child-rearing, or simply to playing with infants, and generally, whether bad health conditions could bring about debilitating disease which would further affect the child's ability to learn. All these factors are shown in the multiple-cause diagram (Figure 5.2).

Longitudinal studies have also been attempted, but their conclusions are often contradictory. For example, Stoch and Smythe (1963) followed the progress of a group of 'Cape coloured' children in South Africa who had experienced protein-energy malnutrition, and a group who had not. However, inter-familial social conditions probably accounted for the differences in intelligence test results that were recorded, for despite apparent close matching of individuals in the two groups, the children with a history of malnutrition had much less stable home backgrounds. It is also worth noting the findings of Stein *et al.* (1972) who examined the frequency of mental retardation among army conscripts born at the time of the 1944–5 famine in the Netherlands. While they could find no relationship between the incidence of mental retardation and the effects of famine, there were significant differences in mental development as measured by cognitive tests between conscripts of different social classes.

In many of these studies the socio-economic condition of the household seems to have a greater influence on the child than insufficiency of food. This conclusion is supported by the findings of some research carried out in Jamaica by Grantham-McGregor *et al.* (1980). This showed that if severely malnourished children were provided with extra mental stimulus in the form of toys, visits and play, they began to gain much higher scores in intelligence tests. Even in the absence of supplementary feeding the group experiencing the extra stimulus 'made significant improvements in DQ (development quotient) in hospital and continued to do so after discharge. By six months they were significantly ahead of the non-intervention malnourished group, and were no longer significantly behind the adequately nourished group'.

We can only conclude that if there were a causal relationship between malnutrition and reduced mental development, it would be a very complex one, involving many non-nutritional factors. Since few of the studies quoted have adequately considered any such interaction of multiple causes, they cannot claim to have demonstrated that any one causal link is dominant.

This chapter could be extended almost indefinitely with other case studies of food-related disability or illness. For example, we could study the many diseases – measles, tuberculosis, cancer – where an interaction with nutritional circumstances is established or alleged. In many instances we would find that nutrition plays a part, but only in conjunction with other factors. Reviewing the extent of food-related illness in the world, it might seem that there were two distinct categories, as follows.

1. There are people whose food intakes are absolutely insufficient, that is below the critical limit of adaptation discussed in Chapter 3, even allowing for seasonal variations in intake. Such people will be at immediate risk of suffering some functional impairment if they have not already suffered it. Their resistance to infection will be low. If they are adults, their work capacity will be reduced, and if they are children they will have stopped growing. There may also be some people whose diet could provide enough protein and energy, but not enough of some vitamins or minerals.

2. There are people whose food intake is sufficient in terms of all nutrients, but whose living conditions are so inadequate that they are exposed in an exceptional degree to infections which may precipitate food-related illness as a result of anorexia or malabsorption, or through nutrient loss to parasites. Irrespective of these risks, an impoverished environment in which adults are overworked may offer so little mental stimulus to growing children that their development is held back.

The policy implications of this are that people in the first category may be expected to benefit from improvements in nutrition, and hence from policies directly concerned with nutritional interventions. People in the second group, though classed as 'malnourished' by some authorities, could only be expected to benefit if there was a generalised attack on poor living conditions. A nutritional approach by itself would not necessarily help them much.

Clarity about these issues is difficult to achieve because the habit of thinking in terms of single causes is deeply ingrained in most of us. For example, one model which is quoted often used to explain the connection between low food production, poor living conditions, disease, and malnutrition is Figure 5.3, in which there appears to be a simple one-way relationship between each factor portrayed. There is only one path from each problem to the next. By contrast, Figure 5.1 shows that there are many different ways in which a child's health may be affected by food-related causes, and lack of availability of food is certainly not cast in the role of a unique cause.

Figure 5.3 reflects the outlook of certain economists who believe that the nutritional status of an individual has a direct and identifiable effect on his or her productivity at work. The assumption made is that 'malnutrition' leads to deficiencies in both mental and physical development. Low productivity is the result, and that in turn leads to low incomes, and starts the cycle off again, as in the diagram (Myrdal, 1972; Berg, 1973; Hicks, 1980; D. Wheeler, 1980).

Arguments of this sort tend to imply that all that needs to be done to break the 'vicious circle' is to raise the productivity of the labour force. This might be achieved by the application of capital

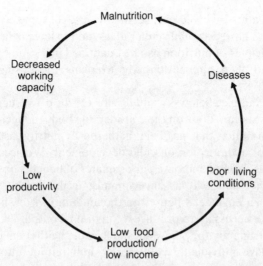

Figure 5.3 'The vicious circle of malnutrition' as it is commonly and simply conceived

and technology, but equally well perhaps by an improvement in the 'quality' of the labour force. For the very poor, inadequate nutrition is regarded as the main constraint to overcome in improving labour quality. Feeding or other programmes which 'cure' malnutrition of the poor would therefore be expected to prevent its recurrence in the future, since productivity would be increased, and the circle broken. Similarly, it has been argued that basic education (especially the acquisition of literacy) can be, 'the best possible means' of overcoming the problems of slow economic development (Rogers, 1969). It is even said that in some societies – Sri Lanka and Kerala have been cited – people have achieved an improved standard of nutrition with a limited food supply because literacy has enabled 'nutritional awareness' to spread (Gwatkin, 1979).

Needless to say, neither extra food nor literacy is a self-sufficient answer. To argue that a single policy by itself is the key to the elimination of poverty, rather than a combination of complementary policies, is to fall into the trap of single-cause thinking. The most fundamental limitation of vicious circle arguments is that they reflect such reasoning. The over-simplification involved may seem obvious, yet some economists appear to have accepted similar ideas, and to have believed that the principles of nutrition can be quantified in a straightforward way and then applied directly to plans for raising labour productivity.

For example, Selowsky and Taylor (1970, p.18) suggest that economists can 'draw on the considerable body of "technological" information that has been gathered by nutritionists on the effects of malnutrition on child development. We accept these results as definite and base our estimates of benefits on them, in much the same way as an economist evaluating a steel mill accepts an engineer's figures on the amount of iron, limestone and coke necessary to produce a ton of final output'.

Unfortunately for Selowsky and Taylor, neither children nor adults have individually fixed energy input–output ratios. As we say in Chapter 3, variability in the body's energy intakes and energy needs is not well understood and the discussions in this chapter should have dispelled any notion that the causes and effects of food related illnesses can yet be quantified in a straightforward way.

These rather simplistic attitudes are the result of an idea about systems which has developed in many disciplines. This postulates an equilibrium situation in which the system is 'optimised' so that it functions in a harmonious way and at a peak of efficiency. If a system (which might be a society, or a household, or an individual body) is seen to be performing badly, it is assumed to be because one or more of its elements is not functioning properly. According to this logic, if we can identify the faulty component and fix it, the system will become optimal again and will then remain so. In previous chapters, however, we have seen ample evidence that this view does not work when applied to the human body. Low productivity cannot be explained by a mechanistic, fixed-efficiency model of human work capacity.

However, we ought also to consider the limitations of vicious circle arguments in a broader context. A diagrammatic representation of the factors influencing problems of the kind we are considering will often need to be a fairly complex network (Figure 5.1) rather than a neat circle. The network will represent various kinds of interaction between causative factors, some of which will take the form of feedback loops. Almost always when a vicious circle is spoken of, a feedback loop is being referred to, but in isolation from other interactions. For example, it is sometimes said that there is a 'vicious circle of low incomes, high birth rates, and slow development' (Rogers, 1969). According to this view, incomes remain low because increases in production are consumed by the increases in population rather than in raising per capita living standards.

However, to use another analogy, there is not just a simple race between population and food production such that if the population grows too fast, poverty and hunger increase. There are several different races in progress – several trains of cause and effect – and this means that several kinds of feedback are operating (Poleman, 1981). At present, food supplies in most parts of the world are well able to keep up with the growth in the numbers of people able to buy food. Many people are eating less food than is desirable, and occupy poor housing with bad sanitation, not because food is short, nor because building materials are scarce, but because there is a real and urgent shortage of 'livelihoods', that is, or opportunities to be employed, to produce, to earn. It is opportunities for employment that are lagging behind population growth, not food production, and it will be part of our task in Part III to explore further the network of causes and effects which limits their expansion.

6 Functional classes and targeted policies*

Identifying the malnourished

There is a long history of attempts to introduce a degree of nutritional thinking into food supply planning by comparing the food balance sheet for a nation with an estimate of its overall nutritional requirements. Policies for agricultural inputs, price controls, and subsidies are then supposedly influenced by what is thought necessary to close any gap between food supplies and needs.

The fallacy involved in averaging nutritional needs over national populations has already been mentioned (Chapter 4). To illustrate further how it misrepresents the condition of a population, Figure 6.1 shows a hypothetical situation in which some people are suffering from undernutrition and some from overnutrition. Curve A represents the distribution of intakes of some nutrient, or perhaps food energy. Curve B is a 'risk function' which shows that at very low levels of intake, the risk of becoming malnourished is very high, and that with large intakes, people are liable to become unhealthy because of 'overnutrition'. In between is a zone of successful adaptation.

The numbers of people in the population facing unacceptable risks are shown by the hatched areas under the 'tails' of curve A.

---

*This chapter utilises material prepared by Peter Cutler, Elizabeth Dowler, Barbara Harriss, Philip Payne and Erica Wheeler.

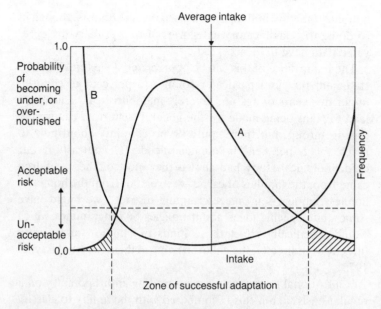

Figure 6.1 Numbers of people with particular levels of nutrient intake (curve A), and the degree of risk associated with the same intakes (curve B), plotted against the actual intake level

Notes: The graph represents a hypothetical population in which under-nutrition and over-nutrition both occur.

Nutritionists and planners will be concerned to see these numbers reduced, but aggregate indicators of food availability do not give any information about them. Policies which influence the average level of demand for a nutrient may or may not change the shape of curve A, reduce the size of the 'tails', or alter conditions for the people they represent.

A refinement would be to seek disaggregated data about separate groups of people, remembering that whether or not a person suffers malnutrition depends on factors such as the ecological setting, the season, the incidence of disease, the domestic environment, the work being done, control over production, the wages received, and the market price for food. The aim would be to understand the epidemiology of malnutrition in terms of its distribution among various ecological regions and socio-economic classes. The disaggregated data from which national totals are built up can be used by nutritionists, though in so doing the classificatory categories of that primary disaggregated data have to be accepted.

The importance of this can be appreciated if we think about a statement that in a particular country '5 per cent of children under five years of age are severely malnourished'. This could lead to plans being made for the general welfare of children in this age-group, but there could be no certainty about how to reach the 5 per cent in greatest need. By contrast, if our epidemiological study had shown that most of these children came from the families of carpet-weavers, or from the homes of landless labourers in maize-cropping districts, we might have some quite specific ideas about policies or programmes which would specifically affect those kinds of families, and, either directly or indirectly, the children living in them (Joy and Payne, 1975).

If nutritional status can be measured by anthropometry on a regular basis, and if this is combined with the ability to classify people – by relation to the means of production (occupation, income, assets) by location, by broad types of product – the resulting information system could be used in precisely the manner required to check on the fortunes of carpet-weavers' and labourers' children. It could also be used as a basis for evaluating the implementation of government policy.

Arguably, then, nutritionists should reduce their efforts to specify global estimates for the numbers of the malnourished, to measure average figures for food consumption, and to setting general criteria of adequacy of food intake. An effective description of the problem of malnutrition requires comparative data, at least as much, if not more than absolute measurements – especially data that are comparative as between social groups. The need is to identify more carefully *who* in the population is malnourished, and *why*.

This is not a Utopian proposal; a few countries have successfully established information systems of this sort using existing data collection networks (Valverde *et al.*, 1981a). In India, the state-by-state analysis of food consumption surveys clearly shows the very low energy intakes of landless peasants and small farmers with less than one acre. Using such information, types of household at risk can be ranked. Population figures can be broken down by occupation and farm size using District Census manuals and agricultural census data. If agricultural and nutritional data for a given State census were collected in this way, nutritionists would even now be able to group and identify the malnourished. At present, many nutritionists are not aware of these data, or of its potential contribution to their professional activities.

It follows that a first stage in any study aimed at identifying those at risk of falling below an established nutritional cut-off point will often be the analysis of existing data on occupational groups and their distribution. It is important that such analysis should precede any new nutritional survey, in order to identify the socio-economic classes which the survey should sample. Too often, sampling in nutrition surveys is random, and any subsequent analysis then has to make do with data that has not been gathered with the purposes of the analysis in view.

What is required, therefore, is a classification of 'the nutritionally deficient population which makes it possible to relate nutritional deficiency patterns to spatial, ecological, socio-economic and demographic characteristics of the population' (Joy and Payne, 1975). This has been termed a functional classification,* and needs to be designed in relation both to the existing data, and the political and budgetary possibilities for intervention.

In practice, a functional classification will vary greatly according to local circumstances and depending on data already available. However, since the aim is to produce results applicable to policy, it would usually subdivide the region in a way that is accessible to intervention concerned along the boundaries of the administrative districts within which policy is implemented. In each district however, both ecological and administrative sub-zones would be identified, and within each one, people likely to be facing nutritional deficiencies would be classified according

---

*In this context 'functional' implies that the classification itself has a function – that of indicating causal factors in malnutrition.

to the availability of disaggregated data. In India, for example, the National Nutrition Monitoring Bureau uses an elaborate sampling procedure to ensure that its coverage within each State is representative of different levels of agricultural development, and different sizes of village. Then within each village, the selection of households for inclusion in food consumption surveys is designed to ensure 'proper representation' of different 'segments of the population, e.g. Harijans, artisans, landless labourers, small or medium land owners and well-to-do groups' (Swaminathan, 1982). Thus, although the NNMB clearly excludes the idea that high nutritional risk is so closely associated with particular agricultural regions or village sizes that surveillance can be regionally targeted, the social sampling does focus on the nutritionally vulnerable (predefined in overlapping categories : caste, occupation, landholding). A survey of households in rural Laguna in the Philippines used the proportion of preschool children below 75 per cent of Harvard standard weight-for-age as a basis for comparing the nutritional status of different groups. This identified the people most at risk as the families of 'small' fishermen, and to a lesser extent, small farmers and labourers (Omawale, 1980). Many surveys disaggregate social groups simply by income, but this study underlines the importance of disaggregating by occupation as well, because the earnings of the small fishermen were by no means low.

In Costa Rica, censuses of population, housing and agriculture carried out in 1973 made it possible to identify a great many occupational groups and to break them down by administrative and geographical location in a very detailed manner. When this was followed up by a nutritional status survey, again measuring weight-for-age, it was possible to see that certain groups of people faced quite severe problems. Among these were labourers in sugar and banana plantations, and farmers growing basic grains and coffee. By contrast, cattle farmers and dairy workers appeared to face few nutritional problems.

Costa Rica is unusual in its large budget for social welfare; its experience of programmes aimed comprehensively to help all the poor goes back to the 1940s. Since then, living conditions for most low-income groups have improved, but by 1970 it was recognised that a new approach was required to tackle pockets of 'extreme poverty' which had so far not been touched (Valverde *et al.*, 1981a; Valverde *et al.*, 1981b). The information system described above grew out of that perception and has become a permanent part of the rural health programme (PSR) whose implementation was begun in 1974. Beside nutrition status, as Table 6.1 shows the information system records immunisation, housing conditions, and latrine construction. Health workers visit households regularly, and continually update the information. They themselves use it in planning work six months ahead; it can also be used in other types of welfare programme. Since these will not always be within the same boundaries as the health work, the data are retained in a disaggregated form in files referring to families or households. Ideally, this will be a standard feature with any functional classification, since it allows information to be re-analysed at any time using different categories.

Other surveys which relate nutritional status to the details of socio-economic conditions are scarce. One example from the Philippines was quoted above. Another is the work in Nepal described earlier; cultivators there were differentiated according to how much land they used. Table 5.1 in the previous chapter indicates some of the differences between the groups so identified. For example, 16 per cent of children living in households with access to less than 0.5 ha were below the defined cut-off level for weight-for-height. The corresponding proportion in households cultivating more than 1.0 ha was only 2 per cent (Nabarro, 1981).

Planning agricultural projects

We begin to see that it is rarely possible for income-raising or food subsidisation policies to be implemented in such a way that they can benefit all the poor simultaneously. Very often, specific measures must be targeted to the most vulnerable groups if these latter are to be reached, without massive implications for budgetary and administrative allocations.

Table 6.1   *Costa Rica: some nutritional and socio-economic characteristics of functional groups*

Functional groups	Fam.	Malnutrition gr. 2 and 3	Average income in colones (C)	% fam. with income < C2100[1]
AW vegetables and fruits*	54	9.3	1033	94.0
AW unknown products	432	9.3	1125	93.3
AW basic grains	165	9.1	738	100.0
AW coffee	975	9.0	955	95.8
Unskilled workers and artisans	415	8.9	1583	82.5
AW beef cattle	70	8.5	1020	95.7
F. from 1 to 3 ha.*	641	8.1	1055	94.4
F. from 5 to 10 ha.	359	7.8	1328	84.7
F. from 3 to 5 ha.	316	7.3	1381	84.8
AW cattle not specified	416	6.7	966	91.7
Workers in the transitory informal economy sector	229	6.6	726	99.0
Pensioners	200	6.5	887	92.8
AW sugar cane	178	6.2	1278	90.1
Qualified operators and artisans	1326	6.2	1936	72.3
All types of management	432	6.0	2363	62.1
Office employees and salesmen	279	5.8	2482	53.6
F. less than 1 ha.	253	5.5	807	97.6
F. from 25 to 50 ha.	199	5.0	1746	78.3
AW banana and african palm	237	4.6	1943	77.0
Service workers	659	4.4	1537	84.2
F. 50 or more ha.	403	4.4	1893	75.7
AW dairy cattle	86	3.5	1266	92.8
F. from 10 to 25 ha.	471	3.4	1290	86.0
Professionals and technicians	333	1.8	4038	12.4
TOTAL	9441	6.6	1514	82.2

Notes:
*AW = Agricultural workers; F. = Farmers.
[1] In 1980 8.60 (colones C) = US$1.00

Source: Family and Community Questionnaire, Ministry of Health, 1980.
Taken from *Social Statistics Bulletin*, vol.4, no.4 (UNICEF, 1981).

% fam. with per capita income < C375[1]	% fam. with very deterior- ated housing	% fam. with crowding gr. 2 and 3	% fam. in housing with earth floor	% fam. with- out domestic piped water supply	% fam. with a deficient excreta disposal system
88.0	31.4	51.0	16.7	64.8	86.8
90.3	24.8	59.8	24.8	53.1	89.8
99.3	38.7	69.7	49.7	57.3	96.8
96.2	17.1	60.2	20.7	40.1	90.8
71.7	16.7	52.9	18.0	25.7	67.3
94.3	11.9	54.7	31.4	60.0	92.5
91.0	12.3	43.7	17.3	44.4	84.8
87.1	8.7	43.2	9.6	65.0	82.6
83.3	9.4	44.9	12.1	47.9	83.1
94.6	19.7	52.3	25.5	67.2	90.9
96.5	32.9	64.4	31.8	57.3	91.9
88.3	23.2	46.2	27.8	29.4	69.0
86.0	21.9	38.8	9.4	15.2	51.3
55.6	9.0	59.8	13.0	44.9	88.1
50.6	6.1	30.4	6.3	17.4	41.3
37.6	4.0	26.7	5.1	10.5	28.1
93.9	14.7	54.6	22.4	45.6	89.2
77.7	8.2	38.2	13.3	60.1	82.8
46.8	8.1	41.5	6.8	30.5	58.0
71.5	15.4	42.8	10.2	55.7	75.4
74.9	8.8	50.1	18.6	20.7	65.1
88.0	11.6	31.4	8.1	50.6	75.9
85.4	11.1	45.9	12.6	63.0	88.8
12.1	1.8	15.8	1.8	8.5	20.5
75.5	13.9	46.4	16.0	37.5	72.0

Similar considerations apply to agricultural projects. We cannot assume that programmes designed to raise food output and income can be implemented equally well by all farmers. Yet it would be possible to identify those who have difficulty in adopting a new technique, and this information could be used in planning local activities regarding such things as credit, fertiliser distribution, or improvements in crop storage (Valverde *et al.*, 1981b). But information dealing with household groups and their nutritional welfare can also be of vital importance in national agricultural planning. The 'green revolution' in Asia and many individual projects have shown that increases in food output can have negative effects on the nutritional status of some of the people affected.

For this reason, it has been suggested that survey methods of the type described in previous pages should be used in the early stages of planning agricultural projects. The aim would be to identify the most nutritionally vulnerable groups, and then design the programmes so that they will benefit to the extent that economic and political constraints will allow: or at the very least, so that any possible adverse effects upon these people are avoided. This approach has been suggested by the FAO Committee on Agriculture (FAO, 1981, 1983), which also notes that there will sometimes be projects in which 'no feasible design alternatives will bring benefits to the malnourished groups'. In those circumstances, if the people concerned have at least been identified, it should be possible either to direct welfare support towards them, or to enable them to participate in other types of project which will generate employment and income and thus incorporate the protection of their livelihoods into project planning.

The FAO Committee arranged for the survey methodology to be tested in six countries. The objective was to identify functional groups, to assess their nutritional condition in terms of the prevalence of malnutrition in children, and to make appraisals of different projects and project designs on the basis of their likely effects on these functional groups which had the poorest nutritional condition. In Kenya, they found that food insufficiency was particularly marked among small land holders with few livestock, and in families where male adults regularly moved to the towns in search of work. In Sri Lanka, a similar survey showed that the 'rural landless and estate workers were the worst off nutritionally', despite a government food stamp programme replacing an earlier rice subsidy (FAO, 1981).

A significant feature of the FAO approach is the way in which it has recognised the multiple causes of food-related disease, and thus the emphasis it gives to environmental factors other than simply food supply. Thus the Committee on Agriculture stresses that, 'the full potential of development projects to improve nutrition can only be realised if increases in food supplies and effective demand for food are accompanied by improvements in such environmental factors as water, sanitation, housing, fuel and communication services'. Thus environmental factors should be recorded during nutrition surveys, and relevant improvements, e.g. in sanitation, might then be included in the resulting agricultural/nutritional project design.

It is difficult to generalise about methods to be used in a functional classification since the contexts in which the approach may be applied are so varied. However, to summarise what has been said in preceding pages, we conclude that the main categories of classification adopted will usually be as follows (Joy and Payne, 1975):

1. Administrative districts.
2. Ecological zones within administrative districts, especially urban vs. rural, and rural sub-zones as characterised by cropping patterns, etc.
3. Economic sub-groups within the populations of the ecological zones, as indicated by income, class, occupation, etc.
4. Demographic categories within sub-groups, e.g., mothers, other adults, preschool children, older children.
5. Food deficiency patterns, e.g. whether they are chronic, seasonal or occasional.
6. Nutrient deficiencies: energy and protein, or specified vitamins or minerals.

The most complex of these categories, requiring considerable further subdivision, might be the 'economic sub-groups'. Here we might need to distinguish between poor people with stable employment and those only spasmodically employed or wholly unemployed. In urban areas, we might need to look at the specific problems of recent migrants, and ask whether they are successfully adapting their eating habits to the food available in their new environment. We will often need to distinguish 'surplus' from 'deficit' farmers, and both of these from the landless and from nomads.

Once a preliminary classification has been decided on, households can be sampled to collect information on nutritional status. But it will also be possible to improve the definition and description of the functional groups in a number of ways. Firstly, besides recording quantitative numerical data on anthropometry, field workers may collect descriptive information about various aspects of the domestic environment. This will lead to 'profiles' (Joy and Payne, 1975) of typical households being recorded with emphasis on food and fuel resources, weaning and feeding habits, food preparation and water supply – and seasonal changes in all of these. This descriptive information will be used to develop models of causality of malnutrition along the lines discussed in Chapter 5.

A second way of developing the procedure will be to use it as a basis for distinguishing three aspects of malnutrition, namely, its manifest, risk and trend components (Joy, 1980). 'Manifest' malnutrition is the immediate and visible aspect, seen in individuals with functional impairment of some kind, and for whom treatment or other direct intervention may be urgently needed. This will most commonly be represented by an indicator such as the prevalence of preschool child malnutrition, but where such data are available, they should also include evidence of the nutritional status of pregnant women, and of other adults – perhaps on a seasonal basis. We will generally find, however, that people in 'poorer' families, by whatever definition, have higher prevalence rates of the manifest condition than those in 'richer' ones. But we will also find that not all vulnerable individuals, even in the poorest families, are malnourished at any one time. Therefore we need to consider the existence of categories of people or families for whom the *risk* of being malnourished is high, even though it may not always be manifest.

Recognition of risk depends on noticing the work patterns and environmental factors which have previously been mentioned. Moreover, appreciation of this aspect shows why we cannot just be concerned with direct nutritional interventions. Reducing the risk factors may well call for improvements in housing, water supply or hygiene, or attempts to redistribute workloads. High risk groups then are those functional classes of the population which have not only the highest levels of manifest malnutrition, but the most significant combinations of risk factors. The magnitude of the 'risk' component is the total size of those population groups.

Developing the capacity of a data system to monitor and to predict *trends* is probably the most technically demanding aspect. It could, however, prove to be highly important in the long run. First of all, trends could be monitored through frequent or even continuous measurement. Monitoring, or continuous surveillance of certain key indicators such as levels of manifest malnutrition, of other household or environmental risk factors, or of food prices, food stocks, or of distress sales of land or possessions, are features of nutritional surveillance and early warning systems in many countries. Relating such data, where it is available, to a functional classification will increase its usefulness as a basis for evaluation of the impact of programmes and for the initiation of emergency relief action. But in addition to this, effective planning depends upon an understanding of how the pattern of nutritional deprivation has changed in the past, and upon some degree of ability to predict future trends.

Long-run trends will be comprised of, firstly, changes in risk factors – how have the conditions of the functional groups been changing? Secondly, demographic – how are the numbers of people in the groups changing over time? What proportion of overall population growth is accounted for by the different groups? What evidence is there about migration between groups and regions?

Targeted policies and household characteristics

Even after identifying economic sub-groups within a population, it would be a mistake to assume that households can be completely characterised by the occupations of their working members, or by income. The point a family has reached in its developmental cycle, and the relationship between its needs and its labour power or earning capacity is also important information. The way in which this relationship changes as children are born to a married couple was mentioned in Chapter 1 (see Table 1.4). Each successive child is one more to be fed, and in addition, the mother's earning capacity is diminished as her household duties increase.

Figure 6.2 presents another view of a family's needs and resources. It illustrates an imaginary household where a couple produces four surviving children. Each child becomes economically active in some sense at the age of 10, and the mother resumes some market activity when the youngest child is 2.5 years old. Overall food needs reach a peak as the two oldest children pass through their late teenage years, and just before they leave to set up new homes.

During the early period of family expansion, it is necessary to increase food supply steadily but without any reliable source of additional labour. In this example, food needs climb at their steepest rate of increase, from 33 to 42 MJ per day, in the two years before the oldest child begins to contribute to production. A family which copes with one or two dependent children might thus start to have difficulties when later ones arrive. Gopalan (1969) has certainly found evidence that, in India, the fourth and subsequent children were twice as likely to be malnourished as those born earlier. It is clear, then, that in identifying families at risk we would ideally like to differentiate households with children under working age from those with older children, or containing only adults. Likewise, households containing elderly people who do not work may also need to be identified.

It is generally accepted that in many populations, mothers and young children are particularly vulnerable to malnutrition, but that, of course, does not mean *all* mothers. In order to specify

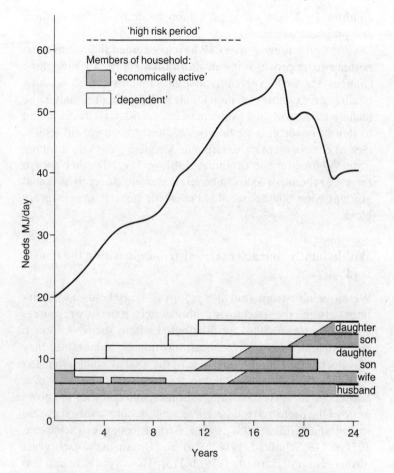

Figure 6.2 The energy needs (MJ/day) of a household for 25 years after its formation (the peak value, prior to the eldest daughter leaving home, is about 56 MJ/day, or about 13,500 kcal/day)

those most at risk, we need to combine information about family composition with the data concerning occupations, incomes, ecology and so on. If this is not done, welfare programmes cannot be directed to those most in need. In India, a crash programme known as the Special Nutrition Programme (SNP) was introduced in 1970. This aimed to provide an extra 1.25 MJ (300 kcal) daily containing 10–12 g protein to women and children. By March 1980, 8.2 million children, nursing mothers and pregnant women were covered by the scheme.

Most evaluations of the SNP have concluded that it has done nothing to improve long-run nutritional status. In suggesting changes, the sixth five-year plan argues that instead of directing feeding programmes at individuals, whole families should be included, because: 'the problem of malnutrition is closely linked to that of poverty, large family size, unemployment, illiteracy, lack of environmental sanitation and hygiene, and safe drinking water' (Government of India, 1981, p.379). To this end, a targeted scheme of loans to generate income currently is aimed at identifying 600 households below the poverty line in every block.

Within family characteristics/distribution within the household

We move now from studying groups of households and variations between them to looking more closely at the way resources and food in particular are distributed within them. Although mothers and infants are seen as nutritionally vulnerable, they may not always get their full share of the food available. In many countries, there are established traditions that the men of a household are served first at meal-times, and that they are given more of the preferred foods such as meat. Examples are reported from India (Gulati, 1981), some African countries (Schapera, 1971, p.143; Schofield, 1974, p.25), and Britain in the early years of this century (Burnett, 1979, p.175). However, although it is often said that mothers cut down on their own food intakes rather than see their children or husbands go hungry, many observers believe that while adult women may end up with a lower quality diet than men, their energy intake does not usually suffer disproportionately (Lipton, 1982; Abdullah and Wheeler, 1985). The one group where there is clear evidence of food discrimination against females is the 0–4 age group, especially in Bangladesh and north India. In Bangladesh, and in West Bengal a 'sex bias' has been found in the feeding of children aged under four, such that male children were more likely to receive an adequate energy intake, and more female children than males were classed as 'malnourished' (Chen *et al.*, 1981b; Abdullah and Wheeler, 1985; Sen and Sengupta, 1983). Data from seventeen villages in the Punjab have similar implications (Levinson, 1974; Lipton, 1982, p.56). In Nepal, by contrast, no differences were found in nutritional status between boys and girls (3–10 years) from the Terai region (Martorell, Leslie and Moock, 1984). The accurate measurement of food distribution within families is exceedingly difficult, not least because the process of measurement itself influences behaviour and makes it untypical. Evidence of the effects of undernutrition on child growth or mortality is easier to obtain but harder to interpret, since exposure to infection may influence the latter so strongly. Nonetheless, when child mortality rates can be disaggregated, they may offer useful clues concerning the epidemiology of malnutrition, and especially the location of families at greatest risk. Child mortality might turn out to be worse in large families than in small ones because of the problems of meeting steeply rising food needs (Figure 6.2). Differences in mortality between male and female children may also be significant. A slight excess of male deaths is usually observed; marked departures from that may imply divergent feeding practices or other differences in child care.

The data for India have recently been reviewed by Dyson and Moore (1983). Child mortality rates are 'decidedly to the disadvantage of the female' in such northern states as Uttar Pradesh, Punjab and Haryana. Sample registration statistics from these states showed mortality rates in 1968–71 that were some 20 per cent higher for females under five years than for males. However, these figures are not in a form that can be disaggregated by district, so Dyson and Moore next looked at the sex ratio of the child population which *can* be traced with some precision through district-level data, and used them as the basis of a rather striking map (Figure 6.3). They comment that India can be roughly divided into two by a line that follow the contours of the Satpura hill range and extends eastwards into southern Bihar. To the south of this line, sex ratios are generally lower than to the north. This difference has been widely recognised in

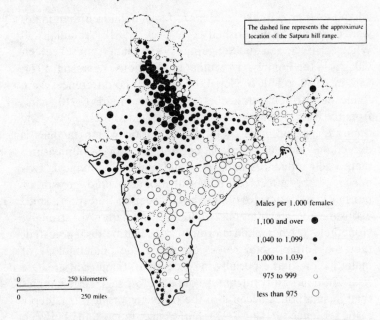

The dashed line represents the approximate location of the Satpura hill range.

Males per 1,000 females

1,100 and over ●

1,040 to 1,099 •

1,000 to 1,039 ·

975 to 999 ○

less than 975 ◯

0   250 kilometers
0   250 miles

Figure 6.3   Sex ratios of children aged 0–9 in India, plotted by district using 1961 data

Source: from David E. Sopher (ed.), *An Exploration of India*, copyright © 1980 by Cornell University Press and the Longman Group Ltd. Reproduced by permission of both publishers.

the past, but is now much better documented, and can be understood in terms of, 'age-old practices of discrimination against females in respect of food and medical care' (Dyson and Moore, 1983, p.51).

Implications for policy: low price shops and ration cards

If it were possible to devise educational, child care or feeding programmes to counter the unequal treatment of female children where evidence suggests it exists, the existence of these disaggregated data would enable resources to be concentrated in districts where the problem is worst subject to the political feasibility of geographical discrimination. Similarly for the more usual kind of nutrition programme, it is tempting to believe that if the most urgent problems could be located within a particular type of family, perhaps in a specific economic sub-group in a certain district, then that problem might be tackled much more directly. However, improving the definition of target groups does not always result in greater impact upon those more precisely defined as recipients, nor does it inevitably increase the cost effectiveness in terms of numbers of intended beneficiaries reached per unit cost of the programme. In practice, there are trade-offs to be considered. Not only is high precision of target group definition costly in terms of logistics (beneficiaries must be identified *and* monitored), but also there are leakages. The direction of benefits to some means preventing these benefits from reaching others, either because of inefficiency or through corruption. Low precision of targeting on the other hand implies the broader spreading of resources, but it also may result in less administrative cost, less corruption, and a much wider sense of social participation.

There are however some kinds of interventions for which a degree of targeting, perhaps simply on a geographic basis seems to be clearly justified. A good example is the siting of low price food shops in Costa Rica. The network of 250 low price shops established in Costa Rica in the 1950s was set up without benefit of an information system identifying areas of greatest need. Thus the shops were located in city districts which were 'obviously' poor and in the more accessible rural centres. Recently, however, thought has been given to opening new shops in rural areas to sell staple foods and some non-food commodities at much reduced prices, and Valverde *et al.* (1981b) have commented on the type of information required 'to ensure that the programme will reach... those families in greater need'. In addition to data identifying concentrations of such families, it may be important to know about incomes, patterns of indebtedness, food grown by the families themselves, and likely seasonal variations in demand, so that supplies to the shops can be planned. 'The most adequate location of the low price shops..and their accessibility for those living on the outskirts of the villages – usually the most deprived – should also be analysed.'

In India, the system of *fair price shops* also grew up without benefit of detailed information on such matters. The service is usually limited to low to middle income groups by virtue of the ration card required to purchase the subsidised food, the cards usually being obtainable only by families whose income is below a specified level. However, the system has various drawbacks, which Harriss (1983b) has summarised. Low-income groups in urban areas undoubtedly benefit, and so do people in some occupations: industrial workers and government employees. But many people in rural areas are not reached by the network and may even subsidise it through the higher price they pay for 'free market' grain. The amount of food sold at the fair price varies with the relationship between 'free market' and 'fair' prices, and fair price sales are sometimes restricted by an insufficient supply of food to the shops.

Taking a more detailed view, we may note that in 1976–7, a *ration-card* in Kerala entitled its holder to rice and wheat, and for a while there was a sugar entitlement also. In her Kerala case-study, Gulati (1981) observed that most families took advantage of the concessionary rice, but few bought wheat because they disliked it and were not accustomed to cooking it. The sugar entitlement was not always taken up either, and Gulati cites housewives who sold it back to the grocer. The ration card could be used to raise cash in another way also. In one family, when the husband was in hospital and money was needed to buy medicines and extra food, his wife decided 'to pledge her ration card with a friend' in return for a loan of Rs. 100. Pledging or mortgaging of cards is believed to be, 'quite a common practice' (Gulati, 1981, p.11), and may be seen as frustrating the nutritional aims of the system. However, there is some lack of clarity about these aims. Ration cards are not issued on the basis of criteria of nutritional risk such as a functional classification might help to define (because rationed goods include necessities other than food; kerosene, cement, sometimes cloth), and the shops can be understood in part as a means of redistributing income. On this view, individuals who exchange the benefits of the system for cash are exercising a legitimate choice about how their redistributed income should be used.

The benefit conferred by a ration card varies from household to household according to how each family manages its food purchasing. One of many merits of Gulati's study is that differences in provisioning between households are clearly brought out. In the family where the ration card had been mortgaged, food consumption was almost certainly reduced as a result. Beside the husband and wife, there were three older children and two 'preschoolers'. The latter went daily for a midday meal supplied under the State government's supplementary feeding scheme. Taking their own bowls, they each received a helping of a cooked cereal/oil mixture supposedly equivalent to 1.7 MJ (400 kcal). The mother was the main wage-earner and bought her breakfast at a 'coffee shop' on the way to the rice fields where she worked. Apart from this, the family's daily food purchases comprised rice (1.75 kg), fish, coconut and spices, most of which were used in the main evening meal.

The cost of this family's food was around Rs. 6 or 7 per day, and absorbed nearly all the mother's earnings, but it could have been about Rs. 1.5 less if the rice had been obtained with the ration card. Another option would have been to buy tapioca, which provides food energy for about half the cost of rice, but tapioca was not used on days when the mother was working because of the extra time it would take to prepare. By contrast, Gulati cites a family consisting of parents with two daughters at school, nearly all of whose rice (0.75 kg daily) came from the fair price shop. They also consumed 0.5 kg tapioca per day, and in other ways were able to afford a rather good diet by making full use of the options for obtaining staple foods cheaply.

Such instances suggest that fair price shops which distribute rationed goods may be of real benefit to some families. In Kerala, there is a good distribution of the shops in rural as well as urban areas (Gwatkin, 1979), but George (1979) argues that those rural people who do not have access to them actually pay more for rice because of the way markets are distorted by procurement for the shops. Procurement from merchants at less than open market prices leads to their making a loss on the grain sold to government. This loss is compensated for by hoisting the price of rice not sold on levy to government (Harriss, 1979b). There may thus be different views about where the balance of advantage lies in Kerala. In the Coimbatore district of Tamil Nadu, by contrast, the coverage of the shops is very uneven, and there is also a striking variation from year to year in how much grain is sold at the fair price. The quantity of rice distributed in a calendar year has varied as follows (Harriss, 1983c):.

1977: 53,450 tonnes (74 kg per year per cardholder)
1978:   6,619 tonnes (9.2 kg per cardholder)
1979: 13,899 tonnes (19 kg per cardholder).

When we reflect that the second of the two Kerala families quoted was obtaining about 240 kg rice per year from their fair price shop, these average figures for the Coimbatore district seem very low. They were exceptionally low in 1978 because there were abundant harvests that year, and needs were less. However, even in 1977, the amount of grain distributed was not high, and further detail from one part of the district – Avanashi Taluk – helps to show why. Figures from fair price shops during 1979–80 show that 94 per cent of the rice distributed, and 30 per cent of the wheat, went to clients in just four urban stores (Harriss, 1983c). The remaining rural stores – some 44 of them – sold a minute quantity. On the whole, then, the system only works with advantage to cardholders in urban areas. Even when fair price shops exist in the rural districts, they do not always offer an adequate service. Yet as Chapter 4 noted, extreme or 'ultra' poverty is often more extensive in rural areas.

It is tempting to draw entirely negative conclusions. The operation of fair price shops is not altogether satisfactory, and the quantity of food they supply seems too small in most areas to make a significant impact on malnutrition. Similar criticisms are made for other nutrition programmes. In India, all the authors who have discussed budgets for, 'a nutritionally adequate, socially comprehensive, public distribution system' end up by specifying such 'massive levels of public subsidy' that they regard it as impossible for the country as a whole (Harriss, 1983b). In Sri

Lanka, one of the few countries which until recently had an adequate and comprehensive food rationing system, ensuring a relatively egalitarian pattern of distribution subsidies have recently been cut back and benefits reduced to reallocate resources elsewhere in the economy.

A more constructive response would be to recognise that in the design and management of targeted schemes, there will always be a problem of assessing the balance between the costs and leakages of highly targeted designs, as compared with the higher resource needs, but often lower operating costs, and greater social benefits of more comprehensive schemes. If our intention is to try to improve the condition of the very poor, then we may well decide that the most effective way is to lobby for an increase in resources to be diverted to broad programmes. But in doing this we shall need to know who are the most deprived, what is their nutritional condition, and why it is that highly targeted programmes fail to reach them. A functional classification and surveillance system will provide the means for this. As we have seen, India already has information systems of this sort in its National Sample Survey (as used by Lipton to identify the ultra-poor: see Chapter 4), and in the National Nutritional Monitoring Bureau (see pages 124–5).

PART THREE

Food and Nutrition Policy and Agriculture

'Karur paushmash, karur sarbonash (for some it is harvest month, for others it is disaster time). The fortunes of the poor move in different directions depending on their exact position in the economic system.'

Bengali saying, quoted and amplified by Amartya Sen (see Sen 1983)

7 Agrarian change and poverty*

Food consumption

Policies for agriculture have usually been conceived and evaluated in terms of overall national production figures and average per caput consumption, without reference to disaggregated views such as those discussed in the previous chapter. The result has been that important implications of agricultural programmes have sometimes been overlooked. Even so, totalled or average figures can reveal some significant trends. Thus Sarma and Roy (1979) examined both FBS and HCS data for all of India in order to analyse changes in production and consumption of foodgrains. They concluded (with provisos about the paucity of data) that the aggregate consumption of foodgrains was falling, and that this trend was not a result of a shift in demand for one type of food to others, but of a general decline in purchasing power, caused by rising real prices. According to consumer expenditure data for the whole of India collected by the National Sample Survey, and on which Table 7.1 is based, this trend is affecting most income groups. If these figures can be relied on, it seems that nearly all groups are getting poorer, but the middle expenditure groups identified here are being affected most.

---

*This chapter is based chiefly on material prepared by Peter Cutler. (See Cutler, 1982a: topics 7a, 7b, 11, 13.) Note that FBS and HCS data are discussed in Chapter 4, where these abbreviations are explained.

Table 7.1   *Proportion of total expenditure on foodgrains and other foods in India for the years 1964–5 and 1973–4*

	Consumers subdivided by level of expenditure			Average for all consumers
	Bottom 30%	Mid 40%	Top 30%	
Percentage expenditure on food				
1964–5				
Foodgrains				
Cereals	53.74	44.10	28.92	37.70
Pulses	5.75	5.96	4.99	5.43
Other foods	24.08	25.24	29.75	27.39
1973–4				
Foodgrains				
Cereals	53.87	46.35	29.99	39.31
Pulses	3.99	4.43	3.78	4.03
Other foods	25.10	28.34	31.86	29.60
Total percentage expenditure on food				
1964–5	83.57	75.30	63.66	70.52
1973–4	82.96	79.12	65.63	72.94
Percentage expenditure for all other purposes				
1964–5	16.43	24.70	36.34	29.48
1973–4	17.04	20.88	34.37	27.06

Source: Sarma and Roy (1979), Table 12, p.25.

Many consumers in the lowest expenditure centiles, particularly in the bottom 30 per cent, must be 'ultra poor' as judged by Lipton's double-80 criterion (Chapter 4). They buy more of the cheap cereals and relatively little of the more expensive ones. Rice and wheat are widely eaten, but the various millets replace wheat and rice to a greater or lesser extent in the diets of the poor.

Evidence from dry regions of south India shows that among

the more prosperous farming families, rice and some wheat may account for two-thirds of the grain consumed, while in the same area, poorer neighbours take only a quarter of their grain as rice, using no wheat but more pulses, and relying predominantly on the coarse grains (jowar, ragi, bajra and the small millets). However, among the poorest groups of all, relatively more rice is used, perhaps because of payments in kind from employers, or because of the example effect of grain distributed through fair price shops (Harriss *et al.*, 1984).

Food production

When we turn from the evidence of falling foodgrain consumption to consider aggregate production, the data from India give a very different impression. The whole agricultural sector has apparently been growing at an annual compound rate of just under 3 per cent since 1949–50. This is quite an achievement by any standards, and needs to be considered in relation to official efforts to promote production. Here we first need to note the Intensive Agricultural Areas Programme (IAAP) of 1961. Out of that grew a new Development Programme (IADP) in 1963, and finally, the High Yielding Varieties Programme (HYVP), begun in 1966–7. It is to the latter that the term 'green revolution' is often applied, and its effects are clearly evident in the figures for production. However, Indian farming was afflicted by a severe drought between 1965 and 1967, and increased production after these dates reflects recovery from that as well as the new varieties (Srinivasan, 1979).

It can be seen from Table 7.2 that between 1949 and 1966, growth in production was fairly even. By 1965–6, there was an average increase of a little under 50 per cent on output of cereals compared with 1950–1 levels. In the absence of drought, this increase would have been greater, judging by the figures for 1960–1. However, in these early years, the foodgrains sector was growing at a slower rate than was the output of some non-food crops such as rape/mustard, cotton, and especially sugar cane (not shown in the table). The result was that the rate of increase

Table 7.2 *Agricultural production indices for India*

Crop	Actual production ('000 tonnes) 1950–1	Index of production						
		1950–1	1955–6	1960–1	1965–6	1970–1	1975–6	1977–8
Rice	20,576	100	134	168	149	205	237	256
Jowar	5,495	100	122	179	137	148	169	208
Bajra	2,595	100	132	127	145	309	221	182
Maize	1,729	100	150	236	279	433	420	344
Ragi	1,429	100	129	129	93	151	196	203
Small millets	1,750	100	118	109	89	207	110	121
Wheat	6,462	100	136	170	161	369	446	485
Barley	2,378	100	118	119	100	117	134	97
Red gram	3,651	100	148	171	157	142	161	149
Tur	1,719	100	108	120	101	110	122	110
Other pulses	3,041	100	124	144	131	156	166	147
Total cereals	42,414	100	132	163	147	228	255	268
Total pulses	8,411	100	131	151	118	141	155	140
Total food grains	50,825	100	132	161	142	213	238	247
Groundnut	3,481	100	111	138	123	176	194	174
Sesamum	445	100	105	71	95	126	108	109
Rape/mustard	762	100	113	177	170	259	254	212
Castor seed	103	100	121	104	78	132	139	149
Cotton	517	100	137	184	159	157	196	233
Jute	596	100	128	125	135	149	134	161

Note:
Index for rice relates to cleaned rice
 Source: Derived from Government of India, CSO, Statistical Abstract, 1978, Table 17.

for foodgrains was 2.87 per cent annually up to 1964–5, compared with 3.47 per cent for the non-food crops. Following the HYVP, this trend was reversed.

Aggregate foodgrain production has been well able to keep up with the rate of population growth, which was about 2 per cent per year over the whole period, but not all foodgrains have shared equally in this achievement. Pulses lagged behind the average level of increase recorded for cereals, and so did the cheaper coarse grains (especially bajra and small millets). By contrast, three cereals stand out as having contributed an especially large expansion in output. Rice production grew to more than two and a half times its original level; maize production to over three times, and wheat to nearly five times its 1950–1 level. The annual growth rate for wheat production has risen from under 4 per cent before 1965–6, to over 8 per cent after this date.

The effect of these changes has been that while rice has retained a consistent 40 per cent share of all foodgrain production, wheat has increased its share from 12 to 25 per cent. This occurred as a result of the 'green revolution'. By comparison, the coarse grains contribute a declining proportion of foodgrain output and this trend has accelerated since the green revolution. The same is true for the pulses, which made up 13.7 per cent of total food production in 1965–6, but had declined to 10.9 per cent by 1970–1.

Generally speaking, for all crops, the increases in total production which occurred before the green revolution came about partly through increases in the productivity per hectare, and partly through increases in the net sown area. There was also some increase in the double-cropped area, which was strongly associated with the spread of irrigation. However, by 1970, the option of increasing the net sown area had been virtually exhausted. Instead, there had to be an increase in productivity per hectare (i.e. yield), if there was to be further increase in output.

Rice, quantitatively the most important foodgrain, illustrates these points well. The area sown to the crop has increased only slowly, from some 30 million hectares in 1950–1 to around 40 million in 1977–8, but cultivators have very nearly managed to double the yields obtained. The massive increase in total output of *wheat* shown in Table 7.2 also reflects a doubling in crop yield, coupled with an increase in the area sown to wheat from around

10 to 20 million hectares. *Maize* yields have shown rapid increases, but have since fallen back, giving a general impression of instability. *Bajra* has followed a similar pattern, with high yield in 1970–1, but lower productivity and also a smaller sown area since. Many of the other grain crops and pulses have made gains in yield, but often with some decrease in net sown area.

In general, then, the HYVP can be seen to have had only a marginal impact on the production of pulses and coarse grains. But it helped other cereal yields to recover rapidly from the bad harvest of 1965–6, and to reach new record levels. To this extent, the green revolution has been successful. Output has increased faster than population has grown, and one might think that people ought to be better fed.

The evidence that average consumption of foodgrains in India is probably falling may seem paradoxical in the light of this. Looking at the food system as a whole, it would seem that increased food production has failed to turn into increased food availability in the average household. In terms of the food system diagram with which we started (Figure 1.1), there would appear to be some sort of dislocation between the uppermost box (food availability in society) and the next one (food availability within the household), sufficient to justify the comment that there has been a divorce between agriculture and nutrition during the green revolution (Palmer, 1972; George, 1977, p.123).

It is precisely here that we come upon one of the most persistent of misperceptions in thought about technology and economics: which is the idea that as long as production is rising, any problems of consumption will sort themselves out. We can begin to see why this is not true for India by considering the strategy by which the HYVP was launched in 1966.

The diffusion of technology

The HYVP was based on the high-yielding crop varieties (HYVs) developed in Mexico and the Philippines under the auspices of the Rockefeller and Ford Foundations. The experience of drought during 1965–7 hastened the implementation of the programme, as did the conditions attached to food aid from the United States. The new crops would probably have been introduced anyway, though perhaps in a more circumspect manner. As it was, the aim was to boost production rapidly, and the programme was deliberately aimed at the richer farmers because it was thought that 'betting on the strong' would avoid spreading scarce resources too thinly. It was also argued that big farmers would produce more surplus for the market.

The key to achieving this aim was the planning of the HYVP as a package programme. Although the new crop varieties were the revolutionary component, they had to be supported by a whole range of other inputs. Irrigation water, fertiliser and pesticides had to be used with the HYVs in the correct doses and at the correct times. If one or more elements of the package were left out, the result could be a yield actually lower than with traditional varieties of seed which had developed the hardiness necessary for rainfed agriculture in a dry country (Chapman and Dowler, 1982). As well as the above technical inputs, credit agencies and co-operatives were revived and expanded to enable eligible farmers to manage the costs involved.

Ishikawa (1967) referred to water as the 'leading input' in the package. With water, productivity could be dramatically increased, even for the traditional crop varieties. Without it, HYVs would produce very little. Therefore, the spread of the new technology was largely restricted to land that benefited from irrigation. In 1965, less than 20 per cent of India's cultivated area was irrigated, but since then, expansion of privately owned tubewells, energised open wells, and government canal schemes has to some extent relaxed this constraint.

Another limitation was that successful (and profitable) HYVs had been developed mostly for wheat, maize and rice, but these were not all suited to local climatic conditions. A few HYVs and hybrids of ragi and jowar do exist, but require an investible surplus on the part of the producer which confines their adoption. The adoption of rice was further limited by climatic factors, and successful HYV strains have only diffused in parts of the south, in particular in Tamil Nadu.

Because many cheap foodgrains, such as bajra and the small

millets, did not benefit from these programmes, they now account for a smaller proportion of production. Declining area and increased demand caused by a substitution of coarse grains for pulses (whose aggregate supply has declined at the highest rate) has pushed up the price of coarse grains bought by the poor faster than the overall consumer price index (EPW, 1979). The green revolution in India has been above all a wheat revolution, and its overall impact on agricultural growth has been limited. It has also tended to increase the gap between rich and poor states in India, because of the bias towards regions where the climate was suitable and irrigation requirements could be met.

Thus by 1980, only about a quarter of India's farms had benefited from the new technology, and those mostly in three or four states including Punjab and Haryana, among the richest (by per caput product) in India. These states have derived much of their wealth from agriculture, and have experienced rapid economic growth. Meanwhile, very poor, populous states like Bihar, Orissa and Madhya Pradesh have benefited very little from the green revolution and have experienced much slower growth rates.

Social change

The effect of the new technology on employment has varied between regions, and is still controversial. It is likely that the new technology leads to an increase in the use of human labour per unit of land, especially seasonal labour, but that it also leads to a decrease in human labour input per unit of production (UNRISD, 1974).

The major outcome, however, is the impetus given by the new technology to an existing trend towards a new set of class relations in the countryside, which we can identify as coming about through a decline in the power of the landlord class and the rise of the 'rich peasant', 'progressive farmer', or 'capitalist'. This should cause no surprise, bearing in mind that the HYVP was introduced in a deliberately selective way. One result, however, has been an erosion of traditional relationships within the rural economy. Some landlords have altered sharecropping and other tenancy arrangements by increasing rents in return for inputs by demanding cash rents, or by assuming direct control over land formerly rented out. The appearance of entrepreneurial farmers employing unbonded wage labour has 'upset the paternalistic character' of earlier arrangements (Byres, 1981, pp.428, 431; UNRISD, 1974). When harvests have increased dramatically, a farmer may no longer wish to pay his harvesters with a fixed proportion of the crop, as the traditional attached labourers would expect, and the value in terms of food of new types of payment has declined in certain regions.

Some debate has taken place regarding the extent to which such changes have led to small cultivators losing access to land. In 1971, more than 26 per cent of the entire labour force in India was identified as landless. However, that still leaves 43 per cent described as cultivators, and some commentators have argued that the dispossession of cultivators is not as widespread as census figures suggest (Krishnamurthy, 1973). Poorer households have often shown considerable tenacity in hanging on to at least some land, but the area retained is often insufficient for them to gain their livelihood primarily as cultivators (Byres, 1981). Their farming has thus been 'marginalised' rather than eliminated, and they have become more dependent on hiring out their own labour. These changes seem to be occurring very rapidly, owing to the termination of tenancies, the loss of trade experienced by some rural artisans, and the growth of population. There are, of course, new jobs associated with the processing and marketing of the increased crop outputs. There are also employment opportunities in industries producing goods for consumption by households whose capacity to spend has been increased by the new technology (Mellor, 1976). But the extent to which this employment in agro-processing, wholesale trading and in the production of consumer goods and services is rural, local, small scale and labour intensive and therefore of benefit to poor, labouring households, is highly controversial. As to other urban employment, formal sector industrialisation has not proceeded quickly enough to absorb surplus labour from agriculture and anyway is not of a character to create great demand for labour because of the increasingly capital intensive nature of modern production processes. And to expand employment in the State apparatus (including the military) is problematical politically as well as on grounds of the efficiency of resource allocation.

As we have seen, however, demand for labour in agriculture at certain times in the farming year has increased. Indeed, the heightened seasonality of farming is a crucial aspect of the green revolution. Excess demand for labour 'in season' pushes up its prices, and labour might therefore be expected to benefit. However, Lal (1976) has found that real wages in agriculture are highest in states which are *not* associated with the widespread introduction of the new technology. The 'green revolution' states, particularly the Punjab and Haryana, have low levels of unemployment but relatively low real wage rates. States such as Kerala and West Bengal have high unemployment rates, and high wage rates, but are low in ranking of per caput productivity, both in agriculture and industry.

The paradox is explained by two developments. The first is that upward pressure on wages is accompanied by a stimulus to mechanisation. The second is that wages are not paid primarily on grounds of productivity, but according to customary rates sometimes based on subsistence minima and in certain states on the basis of bargaining power backed up by legislation on minimum wages. Bargaining is possible only if working people with no assets other than their own labour recognise the class nature of their position and defend their interests by 'class for itself' action (Byres, 1981). Examples where such action has occurred are West Bengal, Kerala and parts of Tamil Nadu, but there is not yet a general development of class consciousness among the growing proletariat of rural India.

In noting these tendencies, UNRISD researchers point out that in societies where serious social inequalities already exist, technological advances leading to increased agricultural output are always 'liable to be limited to those who have superior endowments of land and social status', excluding the poorer majority. The problem is not inherent in the technology itself, but is a consequence of the impact of the technology on inequalities in access that already exist. As UNRISD puts it, we would be wrong to attribute all recent change to the single cause of new technology. Rather, we should think more about the historical circumstances in which it was introduced. Failure to make allowance for the effects of existing inequalities was a major deficiency in the HYVP. It is by learning from this and similar programmes that the FAO Committee on Agriculture has come to emphasise the more discriminating, disaggregated assessment of the people affected which we discussed earlier (Chapter 6).

Social class and market linkages

Here it is worth noting how researchers perceive class structures. Very often, they identify the poorest class either with the landless, or with those holding less than some minimum amount of land which could provide sufficient food for subsistence. In other words, size of land holding has been used as a proxy for class. Byres (1981) believes that this was a reasonable approach prior to the mid 1960s. With the adoption of the new technology, however, the use of land holding as a proxy for social class needs to be refined by factors such as the form of organisation of labour and the means of extraction of surplus. This means that functional classifications may need to subdivide social classes not only by occupation, or type of product and area of land, but also by level of mechanisation. The nutritional welfare of individual members of these classes depends on workloads, time constraints, and other factors which vary even between wage-earners with the same level of income.

In a study of dryland agriculture in India, Harriss *et al.* (1984) used a criterion based on the hiring of labour to define socio-economic classes. Many households covered by the study hired other people's labour when work on their land was at a peak, but hired out their own labour when they were less busy. Over the course of a year, some families were net 'hirers-in'; other households depended predominantly on labouring for others, and were net 'hirers-out'. The latter often had to rely heavily on the earnings of their female members.

Different criteria for identifying social classes reflect varying views of the multiple causes of poverty. Classification by land holding encourages the idea of landlessness as a cause. Emphasis on hiring labour draws attention to low wages, underemployment and exploitation, and raises questions about the bargaining power of working people. But seasonal peaks in the incidence of certain illnesses, aggravated by poor living conditions and insufficient foods, may also be contributory causes of poverty. A full causal analysis of poverty, whether using the diagrammatic approach of Chapter 5 or some other method, would certainly need to take account of all these things. We should notice, however, that some of the most important of them are encompassed by the concept of 'exchange relations': the terms and conditions under which goods (including labour, and the grain needed by labour for survival) are sold and purchased.

The ability of employers of labour to keep wages low is not simply the outcome of market supply and bargaining power. It is also strongly affected by their control over interlocked markets such as money and land as well as commodities, especially food. Harriss *et al.* (1984) found that those social classes which were predominantly employers of labour also had a considerable influence over the market for food through their sales of grain. At the same time, they were less dependent than most people on purchasing food for consumption. They were the true subsistence farmers.

Meanwhile, those who depend chiefly on hiring out their labour were commonly forced to buy food in seasons when prices were high, and had no choice but to work when wages were low. Labourers with land usually needed to sell produce immediately after the harvest, which is normally the season of lowest prices. Their terms of trade* were more disadvantageous than were

---

*The (barter) terms of trade is a concept referring to the relationship through time between prices paid for a given set of agricultural commodities on the one hand and those for a set of non-agricultural commodities on the other.

those of labour employers and the net availability of food to the former classes was much lower than that to the latter.

Exchange entitlements and food

Access to food on the part of the poor can be achieved directly via ownership or achieved indirectly through trading. The latter is what Sen terms an 'exchange entitlement' (1981). He points out that the resources and relationships determining a household's command over food, its food entitlement, can be derived through production (using land and other assets); and by transfers of resources by inheritance, rent interest, etc., or by selling (or hiring out) one's labour power for cash or food and by trading other commodities with or without the use of money for food.

Focus on the first two items in this list leads to the usual emphasis on landlessness as a reason for poverty. Focus on the last two items brings out the points made by Harriss and her colleagues about the purchase and sale of commodities and of labour as causes of poverty. However, in order to refine our understanding of poverty, we need to think of every family as having, potentially at least, several possible sources of entitlement which constitute its 'livelihood'. Sen suggests that these can be envisaged as a 'map' of exchange entitlements.

This idea might be used to help us understand the question posed at the beginning of this chapter. Why is it that the 'green revolution' in India, with its impressive gains in food production, has been associated with static or falling per caput consumption? The evidence that landlessness has increased shows that some people have lost the option of gaining an entitlement by *producing*. The evidence that wages have remained low in relation to food prices in many of the most agriculturally productive areas shows that the exchange entitlements of those who depend on *hiring-out* their labour have failed to grow.

In addition, we have noted that the green revolution has been associated with a move away from production of the cheaper foodgrains, and this may have had the effects of *eroding* such entitlement to food as people have succeeded in earning. On the latter point, Harriss *et al.* (1984) warn us against accepting too readily statements about nutritional status which are based on numerical information about purchasing power. The availability of cheap food varies from one place to another, and in some areas where people have low incomes, exchange entitlements to food may actually be adequate. One dryland farming area in their study in Tamil Nadu, Kovilpatti, was relatively poor and the expenditure on food of the labouring classes seemed low in relation to food they controlled directly. Yet food energy consumption per person appeared to be greater than in many comparable localities, because the high energy food was cheaper than elsewhere.

In Kerala, generally high food prices have been counteracted by a low-cost food crop, tapioca. While rice production in Kerala has increased over the years at rates which are typical of India as a whole – around 3 per cent annually – tapioca production increased at an average rate of 13 per cent annually between 1961–2 and 1971–2 (Gwatkin, 1979). Although the time needed to prepare tapioca for eating may increase female work burdens, some poor families, at least, are growing or purchasing tapioca as a means of making limited incomes provide more food energy (Gulati, 1981).

The aim of the green revolution policy was to increase food *production*; experience with tapioca and our example from Kovilpatti suggests that if the aim had instead been to increase energy *consumption*, a strategy based on promoting low-cost, high energy crops might have had better results. Further, if consumption is the aim, agriculture might be planned not only in terms of food production, but also in terms of the types and social distribution of entitlements generated by new technology for the rural population. The paradox of falling average consumption in an environment of rising aggregate production has come about because the HYVP and its package programme were designed only to produce certain types of food, whereas the relative prices of that food, the employment generated, or the wages earned in production and in post harvest operations tended to be neglected. The result is that success in producing food has been accompanied by a failure to produce an improved entitlement to that food. As UNRISD (1974) puts it, policies should be formulated around 'the goal of improved family livelihood rather than around production targets'. We can redesign the simple diagram of the food system with which we started (Figure 1.1), where there is a feedback loop showing how part of the food energy which people consume must be re-invested through work to obtain more food. Figure 7.1. shows that re-investment is being directed towards two goals simultaneously – producing food as before, but subject to the constraints of securing a food entitlement which exceeds a given threshold level, and of securing enough income to be able to improve their houses and domestic water supplies, to build latrines, and food stores. For we have seen that it is the lack of all these which contributes to malnutrition.

The exclusive emphasis on food production has led towards 'the dissolution of systems of rural livelihood' (UNRISD, 1974), and the erosion of exchange entitlements. The extra food produced enables the nation to reduce food imports or increase exports, but does not necessarily lead to more being eaten.

UNRISD's (1974) survey concludes that 'the organisation of working cultivators and labourers is necessary', if they are to gain from increases in output. That is as true of India as it is of any other region covered by the UNRISD study.

The limitations of planning

Price trends indicate that many foodstuffs and most basic consumer goods are not being produced cheaply enough to satisfy the *needs* of the poor as opposed to their demand, expressed in declining purchasing power (EPW, 1979).

In the late 1950s, India had been encouraged by American aid-givers, among others, to see its problems primarily in terms of food production, and to enlarge the proportion of planned resources which could be allocated towards agriculture. The room for manoeuvre was small because planners have stressed the need for resources for other basic needs: clothes, building

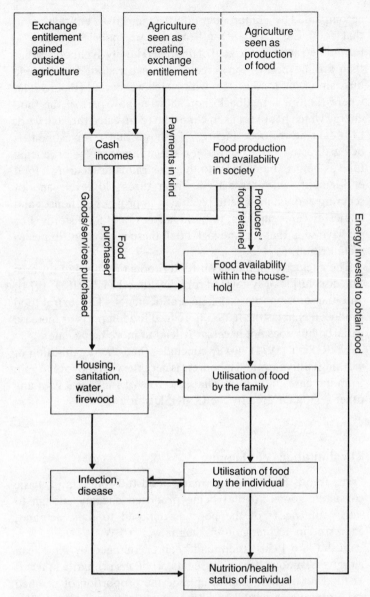

Figure 7.1 The food system described in Chapter 1 extended to include the multiple causes of ill-health discussed in Chapter 5, and the ideas about exchange entitlement presented in this chapter

and sanitation equipment, as well as food, luxury goods and inputs needed by agriculture – fertiliser, pesticides and other petrochemicals – which otherwise would have to be imported and paid for by foreign exchange from exports, or by international al loans.

In India, what has actually happened is that there has apparently been a shift towards the production of agro-industrial crops and expensive food crops with high income elasticities of demand. The result has been what Shetty (1978) controversially calls 'structural retrogression' in the Indian economy. He argues that 'The production structure has moved against the consumption requirements of the masses', and that this development is associated with falling rates of growth in per caput incomes as well as an increase in the relative poverty of at last half of the population. This has been reflected in growing income disparities, which the private sector has both responded to and exacerbated by developing non-essential consumer goods industries. Thus while the production of cotton cloth stagnates, production of toothpaste, beer and cars is expanding fast.

Were it to be established as a political priority that a developing country should concentrate on increasing the per capita incomes of all its people, then India's economy would be expanding production of basic consumer necessities, both food and 'wage goods', at the lowest possible cost. Simultaneously, it would be employing its workforce in the fullest possible manner, so that all its people can earn exchange entitlements sufficient to buy the food and goods they need. Are these goals compatible? In our view this is a key question for anybody concerned about poverty in general or undernutrition in particular.

The emphasis on productivity in planning procedure has led to a situation where those wishing to promote welfare are compelled to argue about people as 'human capital', which will ultimately lead to a higher level of production. Thus policies directed towards proper feeding and education of children are seen as providing investments analogous to investments in machinery. Costs, benefits and rates of return are then calculated in the conventional way (Hicks, 1980; D. Wheeler, 1980).

In practice, however, levels of investment in 'human capital' bear little relationship to labour productivity. People with access to good water and sanitation services, and who live in reasonable houses, may be ill less often than others, but do not necessarily work harder. Those parts of India where productivity is highest, for example Punjab and Haryana, do not have a particularly good record of welfare spending and their productivity cannot be supposed to be simply the result of high investment in welfare.

In an earlier discussion of the 'human capital' theory (page 161 above), it was argued that this was a simplified model which ought to be used (if at all) with the greatest care. For example, to regard nutrition as an investment in economically productive body functions is likely to lead to the view that small body size is an economic advantage, in that it requires less investment and enables people to do certain kinds of piece rate work with greater efficiency. By contrast, while Chapter 3 (page 51) argued that 'small but healthy' people may show effective adaptations to environment, the very existence of these adaptations must often be taken as evidence of impoverished living conditions.

The justification for seeking improvements in nutrition and a related betterment in living conditions cannot sensibly be to present them as 'human capital projects' which will raise labour productivity and break the 'vicious circle'. Rather, they should be seen as part of human rights, to be evaluated by moral and humanitarian criteria. Programmes for the provision of clean drinking water, or primary health clinics, do not need to be justified on any other grounds than those of human need.

8 Markets and food availability*

Exchange relations and famine

Just as long-term undernutrition is now understood to occur because people are too poor to buy food, rather than because of food shortage or ignorance, so also famine is increasingly regarded as an outcome of failure of purchasing power rather than simply the outcome of food scarcity following droughts or other disasters. The dreadful Bengal famine of 1943 occurred in a year when per caput agricultural production was greater than in previous years. A century earlier, food was exported from Ireland while Irish people were dying in the 'great potato famine'. Both instances illustrate a failure in purchasing power or demand. Food was available, but prices were too high, and the poor had too little cash to buy it.

Seaman and Holt (1980) argue that it is possible to think in terms of three distinct but interacting 'observed causes' of famine: failure in the production or supply of food (food availability decline), failure in demand, and failure in intervention. They further point out that in a famine, poor people heavily dependent on markets are most likely to suffer. A slight decline

---

*This chapter is based chiefly on material prepared by Barbara Harriss, with contributions also from Peter Cutler, N.S. Jodha, and Claire Kelly. See Cutler (1982a), Harriss (1976, 1980, 1982, 1983a,b), Harriss and Kelly (1982), Harriss *et al*. (1984).

in food production may cause a much larger decline in the marketed surplus, and can in turn lead to speculation by traders. Then, as prices climb, producers may sell less surplus and speculate themselves, leading to further artificial shortages. The rise in prices of such a basic wage good as food means that people who do not grow their own lose purchasing power over it. So demand falls, and as a result, extra food does not flow into the region. The Bengal famine illustrates this argument. There was government intervention in the market aimed at releasing extra private supplies and preventing hoarding, but it was wrongly timed; the death toll grew to an estimated three million.

Sen (1981) takes as the starting point of his analysis a distinction between conditions that lead to the sudden collapse of food consumption and those that lead to continuous undernutrition. He notes that famine does not affect all groups of people equally, and that some people living in a famine area might not suffer at all, or might even profit from a famine. He explains this in terms of changes in people's food entitlements, referred to in Chapter 7. In an economy based on private ownership of the means of production, where people may be considered to have exchange and ownership entitlements to its products, the individual will possess a set of entitlements derived mainly from paid labour or production, and this may be subject to erosion by rising prices.

In his account of the Bengal famine, Sen argues that there was no shortfall in production, but that the wartime inflationary boom and speculation had begun the process of entitlement erosion. The famine victims were overwhelmingly rural people from a handful of occupation groups – agricultural labourers, fishermen and artisans. These groups suffered because their entitlements were heavily dependent on one base, selling labour in the case of the landless agriculturists, and selling commodities for the last two groups. Market prices for rice rocketed, but their earnings did not. Some poor people did not suffer too badly. These were members of 'economic sub-groups' who produced food crops directly. More generally, people with a diversified set of entitlements were likely to survive.

Markets and malnutrition

Conditions that foster chronic malnutrition must always be carefully distinguished from instances of the rapid collapse in purchasing power which precipitates famine. But the chronic situation may also be usefully examined in terms of the effects of markets on exchange entitlements. Lipton's (1982) review of the concept of poverty, previously discussed in Chapter 4, focuses on the proportion of their expenditure people allocate to food, and thus lends itself to interpretation in terms of people's behaviour in and dependence on markets.

Reacting to Lipton's ideas, Harriss (1983a) has argued that we ought to investigate the dependence of the poor on all types of market, not just their behaviour in one market, that for food. Moreover, we also need some understanding of how imperfect markets are interlocked and might operate to bring about malnutrition.

For example, in a year when harvests are small, earnings from casual labour in the fields or at threshing are likely to be less, but food prices may be higher than usual. If a fixed sum must immediately be taken from reduced earnings to pay a debt, the labourer's exchange entitlement will have been deeply eroded by the interlocking of three different markets – the markets for labour, for money, and for food.

The market for labour might be further distorted in opposition to the interests of labourers by being *segmented*, as when different tasks are allotted according to age and sex. Payment is not necessarily related to productivity, but may be deferred. Smallholding labourers may face choices between more or less immediate returns for labouring for others, and delays until after harvest for returns on labour inputs on their own land. The undernourished are likely to gain a large component of their income from hiring out their labour to many sources of work.

The markets in land and irrigation water might also operate so as to reduce the resources and entitlements of poor people who rent in land. The rent payments may be customary, and may be linked to other markets. They may be paid in kind after harvest when prices are low. They may be paid in the form of labour at times of year when the tenant ought to be working on his own crops. These types of market relationships could operate so as to deprive tenant producers of both investible surplus and essential food.

Wholesale commodity markets might operate so as to discriminate by price, quite legitimately, against sellers of small consignments who present traders with high costs of assembly. On the other hand, lack of transport on the part of some sellers can enable village wholesalers to establish micro-monopolies and make purchases at lower prices than are justified by transport costs to urban markets. Weights and measures may be manipulated. Local and/or illegal taxes may be imposed. Lack of domestic storage facilities may precipitate post-harvest sales, glutting markets and enabling traders to buy at very low prices. The timing of payments due for rent, loans and taxes to the State may also encourage small producers to offload a large proportion of their total sales at one time, leading to low prices. Meanwhile, those producers and sellers who operate on a larger scale can usually keep back a large proportion of their sales until prices are higher. At any given time, the undernourished will tend to be among sellers on to the wholesale market rather than purchasers. They will be unable to speculate. They will be sellers of small consignments of food (grain, also vegetables, dairy and poultry products). Later in the year, they will need to buy back grain and other food on the retail market, when prices are higher.

This argument relating the behaviour of imperfect, interlinked markets and undernutrition requires refinement in the light of evidence. Schofield (1974), examining commodity commercialisation and diet in 29 African villages, found that 'pure subsistence villages are better fed than villages which perhaps oversell their subsistence crops or cultivate cash crops at the expense of subsistence crops'.

For Asia, we have some evidence from a random sample survey of 261 landed households dependent on rainfed agriculture in four districts of south India (Harriss *et al.*, 1984). This evidence relates dependence upon markets of various sorts for income, and net food availability. Unfortunately, it sheds little light on market behaviour and nutrition; this needs special research. When the production and exchange of the sample was studied in 1978–9, some 63 of them could be regarded as ultra-poor by Lipton's double-80 criterion (Chapter 4). Further analysis of this ultra-poor group showed that 47 per cent of marginal peasants were in it, as were 38 per cent of small peasants. Table 8.1 shows that these sections of the peasantry are the very ones most dependent on markets. They derive a significantly larger proportion of their income from 'exchange' than the rich peasants and 'capitalists'. Figures in the table representing net availability of grain summarise the impact of markets.

For example, the marginal peasantry have an average of less than 4 MJ (940 kcal) of food energy per person available each day from grain obtained by their own production and by purchase, and are dependent on other sources for the rest of their intake. They are clearly under severe pressure to find food through labour markets paid in kind (for which we do not have data). Such labouring must provide both small and marginal peasants with up to 30 per cent of their food. The production strategy of these classes is thus nutritionally highly precarious, and their 'compulsive involvement' in markets is evident.

The marketable surplus of agriculture

The existence of markets, especially for commodities, long predates the development of the modern capitalist economy in many countries, and notably in India. Thus market activity is by itself no precise indicator of the level of economic development, nor of relations of production (Chaudhuri, 1979). Historically, peasants may well have been largely self-provisioning, but for over a millennium in some parts of India (e.g. Madras), they have also had to buy, to buy outside their villages, and to sell in order to buy.

The degree of commercialisation of agricultural commodities is manifested by the size of the *marketable surplus*. This term stands for sales net of 'buy-back'. Between 1960–1 and 1973–4, the marketable surplus of food in India grew faster than total

Table 8.1   *Control over foodgrains (cereals and pulses), and dependence upon exchange among 261 dryland farming households in South India*

(The different socio-economic classes are defined in terms of organisation of production. Marginal peasants are predominantly hirers out of their own labour. Small peasants are small-holding labourers. Middle peasant households have an equilibrium between labour days hired out and those hired in. Rich peasants use their own family labour and also hire in labour. Capitalists hire in labour but use little family labour.)

	Marginal peasants (N=43)	Small peasants (N=95)	Middle peasants (N=20)	Rich peasants (N=56)	Capital-ists (N=47)
Average land holding (ha)	1.9	3.5	3.6	7.5	8.2
Production of grain on own holding per person (kg/year)	62	141	178	288	456
Net availability of grain per person, equal to production plus purchases less sales[1] (kg/year)	98	142	160	272	397
Food energy per person represented by grain available*					
MJ/day	3.94	5.67	6.41	10.9	13.5
kcal/day	942	1357	1534	2608	3218
Total income per person (Rupees)	566	645	861	1064	1544
Proportion of income derived from exchange (i.e. from sale of labour, crops, poultry, livestock, and livestock products)	62%	63%	58%	50%	42%

Note:
[1] excludes grain obtained (or disbursed) as payments in kind, and excludes foods other than grain, i.e. other than cereals or pulses.

Source: After Harriss *et al.* (1983).

agricultural output, and foodgrains took up a significantly larger part in the composition of the surplus. This stands in contrast to the position in the 1950s, when the two increased at the same rate, and the proportion of foodgrains in total marketed surplus declined (Mody, 1982). Reasons for this change are not entirely clear, but rising prices and increasing production during the 'green revolution' are clearly important elements in the situation.

A wider perspective can be gained by comparing the long-term development of grain commercialisation in Tamil Nadu and in Punjab. Marketable surplus appears to have been increasing rapidly in both around 1900, but for different reasons. While Punjab was experiencing an increased level of production, in Tamil Nadu about half the marketed surplus seems to have been due to post-harvest distress sales of paddy by small cultivators. The merchant-millers who bought this grain released it slowly on to urban markets, and exported some to Ceylon. But because production stagnated, increased commercialisation depended on a sustained reduction of consumption among the rural landless labour force. This came about partly by paying wages in cash instead of in kind, and by allowing wage rates to fall; partly also it was due to the freeing of attached labour.

In Punjab, production rose as canals were constructed under government authority. Large tracts of waste land were still being settled, and the pressures which might have rendered peasants landless were minimal. Moreover, merchants had less power than was usual elsewhere. They did not control the means of transport. It was bullock carts belonging to peasants rather than merchants which took wheat away from surplus districts and brought back sugar and cotton, or salt and rice.

It was obligations to the State (high water rates and high levels of taxation) rather than exploitation by merchants which acted to decapitalise their agriculture (Mishra, 1981; Calvert, 1936, pp.217, 235). During the period 1908–41, the yields of food crops in Punjab declined and the area under cereals and pulses stagnated. Food production dropped while population grew, and it was commercial crops not consumed locally – rice, cotton, sugar cane – for which production then tended to increase.

The history of Punjab shows that where markets for commodities are not dominated by a separate class of merchants, where producers and merchants are one and the same person, and/or where production credit is not linked to the marketing of commodities, then the process of commercialisation is not necessarily predatory, and also does not necessarily lead to an interlocking of markets. However, we also see from Tamil Nadu that the development of commodity markets may fail to transform production, or expand output when commercialisation results from a change in command over food from those who consume it directly to those (merchants, landlords) who do not.

The role of commercialisation in development

The foregoing examples show that there is no inevitable connection between commercialisation and agricultural development. The former may be a necessary condition for the latter, but it is not a sufficient one. A high level of commercialisation may simply be sustaining a class of merchants which benefits from upward movements in retail prices and pockets the profits, often by controlling the processing of agricultural products.

Nevertheless, trade in food can have an important role in the development of dominantly agrarian economies, and in two respects.

Firstly, price signals representing demand are transmitted through the marketing system so that producers respond with varying degrees of sensitivity by allocating resources to particular crops according to their comparative advantage. That, at any rate, is the theory. In practice, when markets for labour are deeply segmented, or interlock with markets for land, commodities or loans, producers are not always free to respond to the profit motive, and when they are, the price signals they receive do not reflect, even approximately, the need for food, only its demand. Production of a marketable surplus makes possible the purchase of goods not produced by the household. Food may be sold in order to obtain salt or cattle, tools or kerosene, cloth or jewellery. The profits gained in this wholesale trade of agricultural products and this retail trade in consumer goods may then be invested in portfolios of activity which vary according to region in India.

So the second role of a marketing system is to transfer resources *out* of agriculture, making investment possible in industries and services. Physically, foodstuffs for industrial workers (and urban populations), and raw materials for agro-industries are transferred. Invisibly, financial resources are also transferred. Financial transfers may come about via long-term trends in the prices of agricultural goods and of the consumer and investment goods which peasants and farmers buy. Transfers are also made through the payment of taxes and via the accumulated profits of private merchants or public sector trading. While these transfers might often be invested in industry, we should also note that some may be returned to agriculture, or used for 'conspicuous consumption', or in support of the bureaucracy or the military (Byres, 1972, 1974; Nadkarni, 1979). Thus commodity marketing systems are a conduit for resources to flow between agriculture and other sectors. This conduit is clearly necessary, but it can facilitate a *net* extraction of resources from agriculture, which in turn will inhibit the production of food. The nutritional implications of the commercialisation of agriculture must obviously vary with the nature of the process. Hence the means and methods whereby we study this process are rather important.

Evaluations of marketing systems and their policy significance

There are several ways of analysing and interpreting the role of markets in agricultural development. Each methodology has historically been associated with specific policies for the distribution of agricultural products, especially grain. 'Market school' researchers use models of perfectly competitive market behaviour developed in the west. Their general conclusion, which is not always supported by their detailed data, is that foodgrains markets are efficient and play a constructive role in development

(Harriss, 1979a). This approach can only be sustained by ignoring the interlocking of markets, and by an attitude of considerable leniency towards evidence of market distortions. With regard to India, this approach has been applied to markets for wheat (Thakur, 1974; Lele, 1971), rice (Farruk, 1970; Lele, 1971), and jowar (Lele, 1971; Gupta, 1973), and has clear policy implications: the State is regarded as acting inefficiently if it intervenes to replace a supposedly efficient trading system in private hands, and should confine itself to improving marketing infrastructures. This is assumed to make markets more efficient and equitable. It is termed 'market regulation' in India and elsewhere.

By contrast, certain Marxist writings portray the role of traders as a major *cause* of under-development. The traders are said to exert a stranglehold on commodity and money markets, using monopoly power to extract resources both from producers (from whom they buy at 'excessively' low prices) and from consumers (to whom they sell at 'excessively' high prices), re-investing profits 'unproductively' in conspicuous consumption, or else buying land and property with the intention of extracting unearned rent. This also has clear policy implications, the antithesis of the market school: the State must replace such markets by administered, non-market systems of distribution, which will benefit both producers and consumers.

A further interpretation of the role of markets more occasionally encountered in anthropological writing, derives its inspiration from Geertz's (1963) identification of a 'bazaar economy' in Indonesia. The bazaar economy is characterised by a diversity which is not deliberately progressive or entrepreneurial, but which (after the fashion of agricultural intercropping) is designed to minimise risk. Trade is petty in scale, and entry into trade is relatively free. There are few or no modern 'firms', and it has been characterised as 'subsistence trade' (Fox, 1969). Such stagnation in the marketing system is said to reflect stagnation in the productive agricultural economy. Policies to vitalise production will result in an entrepreneurial transformation of the bazaar.

It would be a mistake to regard these three interpretations as mutually exclusive. We can learn something from each of them, and it is stimulating to conjecture that they apply to three different contexts of development. The 'bazaar economy' might be the sphere of circulation of a dominantly pre-capitalist or petty commodity producing society; the trader as agent of under-development might be predominant during the period of the transformation of capitalist production from the stage of domination by merchant's capital; and the trader as entrepreneur might be characteristic of established systems of national capitalist production. Since capitalism penetrates irregularly, whole geographical regions may be at different stages of capitalist evolution. Market towns in transition could possess commodity markets working in different ways. Foodgrains marketing policy would thus need to be regionally flexible. This is very hard to achieve.

State intervention in foodgrains trading

In almost all nations, developed or developing, governments do intervene in private food markets to control and to stabilise prices and supplies, to prevent shortages developing, and with a variety of other objectives. Textbook theory advocates that governments should buy in times of plenty when prices are low (which both reduces its own costs of operation and ought to improve the prices producers receive for their surplus) and to release government supplies on to the market in times of scarcity (thereby lowering high prices and protecting consumers).

State trading could help those vulnerable to malnutrition in a number of ways. If seasonal fluctuations in price were sufficiently reduced, the exploitive effects of interlocked markets could be weakened, because those whose earnings or incomes are reduced at times when the price of grain is maximised would have their purchasing power increased by the lowering of maximum prices; the impoverishing process of post-harvest distress sales and pre-harvest buy-back would be weakened. Table 8.2 summarises a range of government responses that may actually be observed in India. What actually happens is the reverse of the

Table 8.2   *State intervention in food markets in India*

Production conditions	Market symptoms	Interventionist response
Bad harvests	High prices, short supplies.	Rationing, movement restrictions, levies/monopoly procurement, imports, price control throughout the distribution system.
Good harvests	Low prices, abundant supplies.	Relaxation of rationing, reduction of procurement due to reduced sales in fair price shops, relaxation of movement restrictions.
Exceptional harvests	Trend to very low prices.	Price support to producers, exports.

theory of interventions. There are many reasons for this reversal (Harriss, 1983b). Food policy is implemented by decentralised institutions whose financing forces short-term decisions counter to long-term interests.

In India, of the public resources allocated to marketing, the major share is taken by trading by publicly-owned corporations. Before state trading was started, proposals for such corporations were opposed by the 1957 Foodgrains Enquiry Committee on the grounds that they would 'create vested interests' and delay the transition to co-operative control of distribution, which Nehru had envisaged as the goal of social planning. Returns from commercial activities would be directly absorbed by the government apparatus rather than being divided between co-operative members (S.P. Singh, 1973, p.112).

Both with regard to co-operatives and to state trading, there was a considerable development of national institutions in the early 1960s. The National Co-operative Development Corporation (NCDC) originated in 1962 when a Co-operative Development and Warehousing Board split up. Then in 1964–5 the Food Corporation of India (FCI) was set up, amidst controversy, to 'provide a countervailing force to the speculative activity of the trader...to function generally as an autonomous organisation working on commercial lines' (Government of India, 1965, p.2).

The FCI was to co-ordinate both imports and the internal trade, and the legislation which established it also enabled individual States in the Union to set up their own Civil Supplies Corporations. The latter have taken on the function of procuring grain for the FCI according to policies laid down by State governments, and these vary considerably. Thus in one State, sorghum may be obtained by a levy on *producers* paid for at a fixed price; in another State it may be obtained by a levy on the grain handled by licensed *dealers*. Other States may combine elements of both types of purchase, and may also buy a proportion of their requirements on the open market (at a market price higher than the levy price). The majority of foodgrain dealt with by the FCI is wheat (some imported) and rice.

Krishnaji (1975, p.85) has analysed reasons why the official system of procurement offers a much better rate of return to producers of wheat than to those who grow rice. It is possible to interpret it as giving incentives where the potential for production is judged to be greatest, but Krishnaji interprets it as a concession to the regionally and nationally powerful wheat lobby. The corollary is that the lower official rates of return to costs of production for rice evince lack of lobbying power. The same would apply even more strongly for producers of sorghum and other coarse grains, which have probably never been seriously considered as deserving of price incentives (Harriss, 1983b). Such policies neglect foods that are important in the consumption patterns of the poor, concentrating on higher-value crops.

Even so, in the first 10 years of State trading, the proportion of all foodgrains passing through this system was less than 10 per cent of marketed surplus. Therefore, the non-market approach co-exists with the continued operation of 'free' markets in grain of regulated markets, and often of black markets as well. One type of grain may be traded at three different price levels in the same locality. Only in a few States and for a few cereals is the non-market system dominant. Examples are the State monopoly of sorghum in Maharashtra, and the attempt of the Kerala government to implement monopoly procurement of paddy.

Instead of supplying the free market in order to reduce price fluctuations, grain procured by or on behalf of the FCI is mainly distributed through fair price shops at a fixed price. This may help some victims of interlocking markets, but many of them in rural areas do not have a fair price shop within reach. For state trading to have a stabilising effect on prices it would be necessary for official purchases to be made in a competitive market, so that prices throughout the system would respond. We have noted many obstacles to competitive trading, however, and a levy price that differs from the market price. One must also doubt whether effective control can ever be practicable while procurement prices are fixed at the same level over whole States or even nationally.

We may conclude that government intervention in markets for food in India has not so far offered any real answer to the tendency of these markets to deepen and perpetuate poverty by interlocking with other markets, especially those for labour and loans. One further aspect of the State trading system merits more detailed examination: this is food processing.

State intervention in food processing

In the 1960s there was concern about the supposed inefficiency of the rice hullers used widely in India by millers in the private sector. Ford Foundation consultants suggested an automated package of pre-milling and milling machines which became known as the Modern Rice Mill or MRM (Faulkner *et al.*, 1963). One such mill was capable of processing three tonnes of rice per hour, and its cost (with associated grain storage facilities) was estimated as Rs. 2 million (about US$200,000). This size and level of investment ruled out widespread adoption by the private sector, and made it necessary to introduce the package through the FCI and the National Co-operative Development Corporation (NCDC).

In 1970, under the Rice Milling Amendment Rules, an attempt was made to enforce a less ambitious form of modernisation in private mills by insisting that the traditional rice hullers should be replaced by shellers (either of the rubber roll or emery disc variety). Later financial incentives to improve pre-milling processing were offered by government. Despite the fact that licences could be withdrawn from mills that did not modernise, the spread of sheller technology has been confined to a few regions. Elsewhere the supposedly out-dated huller has remained the mainstay of the industry. Indeed, the number of hullers throughout India increased from less than 10,000 in 1963 to 83,600 registered and licensed in 1974 (NCDC, 1975).

These experiences suggest that despite official criticism, the traditional rice huller has proved in practice to be an appropriate milling technology in much of India, and Harriss (1979b) has shown why. Compared with the huller, the MRM employs between three and five times more capital and more than twice as much energy from non-animal, non-human sources to process a given quantity of rice. If operated at capacity, MRM would draw rice from a very large area, and in practice its capacity tends to be under-utilised.

Nutritional aspects of processing

In order to explain why public resources were committed to a technological package which was not cost effective, we must look at the consultants' original recommendations to the Indian government, which were particularly concerned with the impact of the technology on food supply. The consultants believed that much rice was lost through the 'inefficiency' of the traditional huller. They also commented that 'loss in storage is 10 per cent of marketable surplus'. Nearly all the paddy they had seen, 'in farmers' compounds, co-operative go-downs and millers' go-downs had been damaged by insects, rodents, birds and moisture' (Faulkner *et al.*, 1963, p.10). They believed that a reduction in losses would increase food supply and improve nutrition, an argument questioned in earlier chapters. Be that as it may, they were therefore attracted into advocating a package of post-harvest technologies and recommended that farmers be encouraged to sell paddy immediately after harvest for bulk storage in concrete silos which were to be part of the MRM package. Though policies on technology and on trading were conceived in isolation from each other, such a technological arrangement would be suitable for large-scale state trading.

In fact, the estimate of paddy lost in storage made by the consultants was little more than a guess, and is probably much too large. Two careful studies of farm storage of paddy in India have come up with average figures for grain lost to rodents, mould and insects of 4.7 per cent (Willson, 1970; Khare, 1972; compare Greeley, 1978). In 1978, average losses of all grains in the large-scale storage facilities operated by the FCI were estimated as between 3 and 4 per cent, though this figure includes pilferage as well as deterioration and infestation (Chawla, 1978, p.33; Harriss, 1983b). Thus the bulk stores at MRM factories would have to perform substantially better than the FCI average if they were to offer a significant gain over farm storage. But in fact there are reports of fermentation of paddy inside the silos and difficulties with fumigation which cast doubt on whether this high performance is being achieved.

With regard to the milling process itself, the essential tasks are to remove husk from the paddy and bran from the grain, but this may be done either with the paddy raw, or after it has been parboiled (Table 8.3). There is considerable nutritional advantage in parboiling before milling. For one thing, gelatinisation of starch during parboiling hardens the grain so that it stands up to milling better and less is broken. Secondly, parboiling produces a more even spread of B-vitamins through the grain, reducing their concentration in the outer layers, so losses of these vitamins during the removal of bran are less. Table 8.3 emphasises the improvement in B-vitamin content of polished rice achieved by parboiling.

Traditional parboiling entails soaking the paddy in cold water for up to three days before boiling or steaming it, after which the paddy is sun-dried prior to storage or milling. Part of the MRM package was a striking technological improvement in the process pioneered by the Central Food Technology Research Institute at Mysore. Paddy is soaked in hot water at 65 to 75°C (or in saturated steam) for only two or three hours. This practice

Table 8.3 *Milling processes in relation to B-vitamins and protein content of rice*

	Rice produced by milling **Raw Paddy**	Rice produced by milling **Parboiled Paddy**	**Brown Rice** retaining bran
Milling processes	Dehusking paddy; pearling and polishing to remove bran	Parboiling paddy; drying, dehusking and polishing	Dehusking paddy
Degree of polish (proportion of bran removed)	60 – 80%	60 – 80% (40% for some rice supplied on ration, e.g. in Sri Lanka, but this is generally not acceptable on the market)	< 10%
Rice output from 100kg of paddy (i.e. Outturn)	55 – 72 kg varying with equipment and rice quality	58 – 72 kg varying with equipment and rice quality	up to 80 kg
B-vitamins (μg/g)			
Thiamine	0.8	2.57	4.2
Niacin	18.1	39.8	47.2
Pyridoxine	4.5	no data	10.3
Pantothenic acid	6.4	no data	17.0
Riboflavin	0.26	0.36	0.53
Protein (per cent by weight)	7.6	7.8	8.3

Sources: Harriss (1976), pp. 164–6, 168, 172–3; and for nutritional data, Parpia and Desikachar (1969), p. 84.

eliminates bacteria whose activity results in unpleasant smells with the traditional method applied to large batches. This part of the new technology has been relatively successful.

A problem with this method in its MRM version is the high capital cost. However, in the private sector, the process has proved to be adaptable to the small, husk-fired parboiling tanks, kettles and drums of the traditional mills. Indeed, in the North

Arcot district of Tamil Nadu, this locally modified innovation is already widely diffused (Harriss, 1977).

After steaming, in the MRM technology, the paddy is mechanically dried to avoid the uncertainties of the sun and attack by birds. This has proved very unsuccessful even though costly oil-fired driers have been replaced by husk-fired driers. The alternative – sun drying – is not without costs. Although sunshine is a free good, sun-drying requires investment in a drying floor and in the variable costs of labour and maintenance. However, comparative economic analyses of this method and of mechanical drying had apparently not been done prior to the introduction of the MRM.

Another nutritional aspect of choice of technique is the outturn of different types of mill. When 100 kg of paddy are milled to produce highly polished rice, some 28 kg of husk and bran must be removed, and the amount of rice produced cannot exceed 72 kg. In practice, however, some rice gets mixed with the bran, especially broken grains, so 100 kg of paddy may appear to yield as little as 55 kg of usable rice. The traditional huller has been thought of as out-dated and inefficient chiefly because its outturns of *raw* rice were low (in the region of 60–66 per cent) compensating with more broken rice. The MRM package was claimed to have a significantly improved performance, offering the prospect of recovering more rice from the *parboiled* paddy with much less broken grain. The value of the rice so saved would supposedly repay the capital cost of the MRM 'in one year', and the rice would increase food supply (Faulkner *et al.*, 1963, p.19).

However, these claims were misleading and were based on a misinterpretation of the social culture of rice in India. Lele (1970) points out that Indian society demands broken grain for certain culinary preparations. Many rice retailers in Tamil Nadu sell brokens at three-quarters the price of head rice. There is also a high demand for brokens from the poorer sections of society who may be denied rice or millets by local scarcities or high prices, and who will not have sufficient purchasing power for head rice in the foreseeable future. Moreover, most millers in south India sieve the by-products either mechanically or by hand. When this is done, almost the full 72 kg of rice expected from 100 kg of paddy may be recovered, however low the outturn figure recorded for the huller or sheller used. Furthermore, when comparisons are based on parboiled rice in *both* cases, the difference in outturn between the two technologies is only 1–2 per cent.

Public policy towards groundnut oil processing has embodied similar contradictions. On the one hand, the village oil industry is protected, with government loans offered in 1980 for the improvement of the bullock-driven *chekku* or *ghani* (a wooden pestle-and-mortar device) by provision of a motor drive. But on the other hand, public resources have been allocated to very large oil mill complexes and to solvent extraction plants (which process rice bran as well as groundnut oilcake). As with the MRM, the level of investment involved is beyond most of the private sector, and depends on such bodies as the National Co-operative Development Corporation (NCDC).

As with rice, part of the justification for introducing the large-scale technology relates to the reduction of waste. Some oil is left in the cake processed by the *chekku*. In fact this is not 'wasted' since it benefits the bullocks to which the cake is fed. Meanwhile, one of the problems associated with the large-scale plant is the waste through the loss of material in transit and in processing, amounting to 6 or 7 per cent in one solvent extraction factory in Orissa State (NCDC, 1980, p.85). These kinds of losses, characteristic of real world conditions do not get considered in appraisals of technology for the obvious reasons that they are hard to calculate and reduce the appeal of new technology. There is a widespread attitude in government that the technology ought to be used because it is available (Harriss and Kelly, 1982, p.19; Kelly, 1981). As in agricultural research, there is pressure to facilitate the transfer of technologies developed in Europe and North America (see Chapter 10). Those responsible tend to be uncritical of 'modern' equipment and methods which seem 'technically sweet'. The NCDC has links with the Co-operative League of the USA and its programme for transmitting, 'the experience of the US oilseed processing co-operatives' (NCDC, 1980), especially experience of oil extraction, and of quality control based on laboratory testing.

Questions about whether such technology is needed in India tend not to be asked. What is clearly stated, however, is the need for the US industry to find new markets (McQueen, in NCDC, 1980); one is reminded of alleged links between the Indian wheat lobby and US wheat interests (George, 1980, p.63).

We argued in Chapter 7 that agricultural development should be oriented towards the creation of livelihoods, not just production. This is a different sort of nutritional aspect to food processing from the food supply arguments originally and misguidedly applied to justify new agro-processing technology. Are livelihoods preserved and/or new livelihoods created with the introduction of 'improved' technology?

Consider traditional rice hullers in south India. They are manned by an owner (plus family or partners) with between one and six 'technicians' who supervise the machinery, the parboiling and the drying of paddy. There is also a gang of casual coolies, mostly women, who turn the paddy as it sun-dries and who sieve residues, with some men carrying and loading. In a rural area in which some thirty hullers are at work, their output might typically be 8160 tonnes of rice per annum. They will create livelihoods for roughly 30 owners/managers, 60 salaried employees, and 300 (female) coolies.

Suppose, now, the hullers were replaced by one MRM. Working at the rates which currently obtain in India, this would process the same amount of rice in a year, and would create jobs for 28 administrators and qualified engineers, 68 technically-trained employees, and 90 (male) coolies (Harriss, 1979). This supports Timmer's (1974) conclusion about the rice marketing of Java, and the views of Simmons (1975) and Ngoddy (1976) on food processing in Nigeria, namely, that small gains in technical performance are usually achieved only at the expense of the most vulnerable segments of society who most need employment, in this case female labour.

There are probably no good technical reasons why this should be so. There is nothing in the logic of engineering science to prevent machines being devised which improve outturn of rice, use fuel more economically, and give better return on capital, but which protect livelihoods at the same time. What does prevent such machines being devised is the institutional framework within which engineering science is practised. Researchers, engineers and economists work to their own professional norms and their own criteria of what is technically worth doing. The multiplication of parastatal corporations allows decisions and actions to be compartmentalised so that policies centred on welfare goals, professional interests and international commercial pressures can all be pursued without the contradictions between them being acknowledged.

It is clear who gains and who loses. Food markets tend to favour rich peasants rather than marginal ones, dealers rather than producers. Public procurement is at prices which penalise wheat producers less than rice producers, and both less than coarse grains producers. Public distribution tends to favour those who live in urban rather than rural areas, and who work in industry or in the bureaucracy rather than in agriculture. In grain processing, the beneficiaries of public investment are a small number of educated employees of the bureaucracies and corporations; they are also manufacturers of machinery, contractors, merchant-industrialists who control profitable technology, and operate on contract, foreign commercial interests, and international advisers. The losers are inarticulate, uneducated, unorganised, unskilled women.

9 Nutrition interventions*

Agendas for nutrition intervention

According to our previous arguments, there has been a 'divorce' between nutritional welfare and agriculture. Production of a limited range of foodgrains has risen steeply in some parts of the world as improved high-yielding varieties are introduced, yet the prevalence of malnutrition has seemed to worsen. The policy issues this raises may be confronted in different ways, depending on whether one believes that the purpose of agriculture is chiefly production, or whether one sees it more as the sustaining of livelihoods.

The deficiencies of an emphasis on production involve the fact that benefits do not automatically trickle down to the poorest, not least because of their position in the segmented, interlocking market relations, discussed in the previous chapter. But elements of nutrition policy still seem to be framed in the belief that the food consumption of the poor will rise as production increases. For instance, supplementary feeding may be thought of as a stopgap for use until 'trickle down' begins to occur.

Other nutrition interventions may be intended to encourage or enable people to use more of the foods whose production is rising. For example, where production increases have chiefly

---

*Much of this chapter, excepting the introductory paragraphs, is based on material prepared by Erica Wheeler; see Wheeler, 1982.

affected food that people are not accustomed to cooking and eating, then it is often regarded as the job of nutritionists to find ways in which the food can be used, and generally to seek acceptance for it. As soya bean output has increased worldwide particularly in the USA, much propaganda has been put out about the high protein content of soya. Nutrition projects in parts of Africa, Bangladesh and elsewhere have been built around the use of soya foods (Pacey, 1978), and new recipes incorporating them have proliferated.

In India, the biggest production increases have been in wheat, and one can easily gain the impression that food and nutrition policies have been biased towards ensuring that more wheat is consumed. A larger volume of wheat is handled by the Food Corporation of India than any other cereal, despite the fact that rice is still much more important in consumption terms, and sometimes considerable efforts are made to persuade people to purchase wheat. For example, in Maharashtra and West Bengal there have been occasions when it was made obligatory for people who purchased rice in fair price shops to buy some wheat there as well (Lele, 1971, p.231). The consumption of wheat is also affected by international pressures. The 1982 report of the organisation representing US wheat growers' export interests, the US Wheat Associates, contained the following reference to India: 'It is US Wheat Associates' goal to maintain market promotion and technical assistance programs...as they provide an invaluable link in pressurising the (Indian) government to import wheat to complement their own indigenous production.' One of their target groups is the 'rice consuming production of southern India' for which they have developed a push-cart portable bread oven (Spitz, 1983, pp.7–8).

Targeted interventions on the agenda

Not all programmes are so blatantly biased as these, nor are they based on simplistic assumptions about the nutritional benefit of increased production. The new nutrition agenda emphasises the targeting of food interventions. If the purpose of agriculture is seen as to sustain livelihoods, production is still vital, but it falls into place alongside other priorities, such as the need to give people work and use their skills. If the same view is extended to other economic activity, then the concern of the nutritionist becomes centred on people, not on what they produce, and in particular, he or she is concerned with livelihoods that are inadequate or at risk because they tend to lead to malnutrition. To this end, the 'functional classification' described in Chapter 6, or the procedures in the new FAO manual (FAO, 1983), may be used to distinguish between different kinds of livelihood, and nutrition interventions will be targeted much more carefully to groups at risk of passing under thresholds of adaptation.

Responding to mounting rural distress as well as to mounting buffer stocks of grain, the Government of India launched a major *food-for-work* programme in 1977. At least 50 per cent of wages paid in this programme were meant to be in the form of grain. In 1978–9, some 286 million man-days of work were provided and 2.5 million tonnes of foodgrain were distributed (Government of India, 1980). Balaji and Ramachandran (1980) studied the implementation of the programme in two drought-prone districts of Tamil Nadu, and among other criticisms, pointed out that work was provided mainly at times in the year when opportunities for employment in agriculture were at their peak. Seasons of peak demand for labour in rural areas often coincide with periods of food shortage or high food prices prior to the main harvest. In Tamil Nadu, high food prices occur in November and early December. Thus if the programme's chief aim was to provide food, its timing may have been more relevant than it at first sight appears. Alternatively, or additionally, the timing may reflect a need to get rid of excess buffer stocks of grain prior to their being replenished after the new harvest.

Similar issues arise in other countries where public works schemes have been used as a means of distributing food (Jackson, 1982; Wijga, 1982). Not only is the timing of the work often inappropriate to objectives, but in the absence of any attempt to transform agrarian production relations, the earthworks, canals and roads they create tend to benefit landlords, big farmers and transport contractors more than they benefit the poor.

While admitting all these deficiencies, Chambers and Maxwell (1981) make a limited case for continuing with food-for-work. They point out that the food distributed is important in some places, citing the cases of certain workers in south India and Morocco who derive, respectively, 40 and 65 per cent of their income this way. They point out that opportunities exist for making the schemes more efficient and for using them to carry out drainage, sanitation and water supply works which, we have noted, are often needed to complement better nutrition if improvements in health are to be attained.

Where international grain surpluses are disbursed as 'project food aid' in targeted nutrition interventions, the result may be a shift in consumption from locally grown grain to an imported product promoted by the kind of powerful international lobbies described on p.185. In 1979, some 60 million people are said to have received some food from United States sources in this way. Most of it was grain distributed via the World Food Programme or via agencies such as Catholic Relief Services and CARE.

Quoting these facts, Jackson (1982) argues that few of the programmes have any impact on malnutrition. Many people receiving this aid often are not demonstrably malnourished, and in any case may use the food as a substitute for their own purchases, i.e. they simply spend less on food they would otherwise have bought. It could be argued that the food received has been used very reasonably as an extra resource, freeing cash for other purposes. Whether or not overall household consumption actually increases as a result of food distribution is controversial – evidence points both ways. However, the distribution agencies referred to above are often concerned a) that *particular* people should get the food (namely children and sometimes mothers) and b) that dietary *quality* should improve, i.e. the foods given out (skimmed milk powder, wheat/soya blend mix, and sometimes oil) are thought to have a value in themselves in combating malnutrition. Enough was said in earlier chapters to question these objectives. The reader is recommended to other authors for further discussion (Stevens, 1981).

In some countries, prices have fallen and local agricultural production has been depressed. Referring to West Africa, Jackson (1982, p.87) cites instances where food aid projects have discouraged husbandry of local food crops, and have led farmers to concentrate more on cash crops.

However, most so-called 'targeted' interventions have not, in fact, been directed towards vulnerable groups with any precision. It is extremely costly to target a feeding programme at mothers and children in general. Knowledge about which groups among them are most at risk may lead to tighter targeting and perhaps to reduced operating costs if the new target is less spatially diffuse. Many mother-and-child feeding programmes are rather undiscriminating about the economic sub-groups they hope to reach. They may screen potential 'clients' using anthropometry; this is usually done without combining the evidence of manifest malnutrition which this provides with evidence of risk drawn from a justified 'functional classification' of occupational, economic or environmental conditions. But it can be argued that untargeted or minimally targeted interventions are less vulnerable to capture by the excluded, who in cases considered here, will be the well nourished elites.

Supplementary feeding schemes

One major review of 200 such schemes for preschool children was made for the United Nations by George Beaton and Hossain Ghassemi (1979). This showed that in India, though not in all the countries studied, there have been significant increases in heights and weights of children in 'supplemented' groups. For instances, in the Tamil Nadu nutrition project, a supplement amounting to about 1.5 MJ per day was provided in the form of CSM milk and sugar, and the evaluation report states that small increases in children's heights were found. In the Narangwal programme, also in India, the mortality rate among 1–2 year old children fell from 23 to 11 per thousand in response to the feeding programme, and from 23 to 8 with a combined package of feeding and health care, which seems a positive result. More generally, Beaton and Ghassemi found that the benefits of feeding schemes were greatest among the most severely malnourished. If such schemes could be targeted and implemented so as to serve those most at risk, they could be much more effective.

But, the measured benefit of most programmes was anthropometric improvement, and this was surprisingly small. Recurrent illness and accompanying anorexia probably hindered some children from taking the food that was offered. This supports FAO's emphasis on tackling environmental as well as nutritional problems, for without some reduction in the incidence of infection, the number of children who fail to benefit from extra food availability will always be large. Beaton and Ghassemi say that the highest average rates of *extra* weight gain reported from feeding programmes are about 1 kg/year. A generous estimate of the energy cost of this would be something less than 0.1 MJ (or about 20 kcal) per day, which is 'a relatively small fraction of the supplementary energy apparently reaching these children....'

In other words, children do not appear to grow as fast as would be expected if the additional food were used solely for weight gain. This could be explained *theoretically* by saying that the children's level of activity changes, or that their metabolic rate increases, or by finding errors in the calculation of energy inputs and outputs. Or it could be explained *operationally* by arguing that the food supplement does not actually reach the child's family, or is not consumed by the child.

Beaton and Ghassemi's review ends with the comment that current food distribution programmes are in any case 'much too small' in most cases 'to have a major impact on total communities or countries'. This again underlines the importance either of identifying more precisely the groups which could benefit, and ensuring that they are reached, or of securing sufficient budgetary resources to implement nutrition interventions with minimal social targets, with maximum coverage over space and through time and combined with a benefit of sufficient size to be likely to result in improved nutritional status regardless of 'leakages'. The

Noon Meals Scheme in Tamil Nadu, administered to 6.5 million children, is an example. It is minimally targeted to children aged 2 to 10 registered in nurseries and schools. It covers the entire state 365 days a year. It provides employment to about 200,000 women about a quarter of whom are harijans. It provides a larger calorie input than have other schemes (410 kcals/day per child under 5 and 510 per child over 5). Unfortunately data on nutritional status are currently inadequate for an evaluation of nutritional benefit to participants, but it has had a major impact upon the food economy, necessitating an increase in the volume of, and the subsidies for state trading, and increased grain allotments from Central Government.

In conclusion, whether it is fair price shops, feeding program-mes or food-for-work that is being planned, attention needs to be directed to the social and geographical distribution, and to the economic sub-groups from which 'clients' are recruited and/or to the budgeting implications of expanding the target and the employment created by the intervention. Because it is primarily livelihoods that are in question, our classification of potential beneficiaries will be derived from data that relate directly to occupation, labour markets, and markets for food.

Nutrition education

The shift from a production-oriented view to an approach focused on livelihoods makes a difference to the way we think about nutrition education. The purpose of nutrition education is usually seen as to impart information that will influence food choice. But an alternative approach is possible in which an understanding is first sought about how people's food choices arise from their means of livelihood.

A mother, or whoever else takes responsibility for household provisioning, makes choices on behalf of her family which may be regarded as influenced by three factors: 'attitudes', 'know-ledge' and 'practicality' (Church, 1977). In comparing the food choices of one economic sub-group with another, we may find that 'practicality' accounts for most of the differences observed, since this refers to what can be afforded, and to the way limitations are imposed by the family's resources and the constraints on time available for food preparation. Indeed, it has been said that an understanding of how people may free themselves from poverty is not to be found in the analysis of family food choice itself, 'but in the analysis of systems of constraint that limit choice' (White, 1980, p.23).

As to the 'attitude' and 'knowledge' aspects of food choice, much conventional writing on nutrition implies a peculiarly negative view of rural societies. It is often suggested that lack of knowledge is a major constraint, and that people become malnourished because of 'ignorance'. Similar assumptions were at one time made about agriculture, but it is now appreciated that farmers are often very knowledgeable and use their knowledge to make good decisions about which crops to grow on which soils and about planting dates, intercropping, costs and pest control (see Chapter 10). With regard to food and nutrition, there is much less published information about rural people's knowledge, though it is recognised that in some countries, there is much nutritional wisdom incorporated in local teaching practices, recipes and in traditional uses of some vegetables (including wild ones) (Church and Doughty, 1975; Doughty, 1979). Where eating habits are changing, older women are the usual repositories of knowledge about such traditions (Pacey, 1978). The system of explanation for such feeding practices may be different from ours. It may no longer be practicable to use the old recipes. But the knowledge on which they are based may be applicable in other ways, perhaps in improving the intelligibility to local people of a 'dialogue' on nutrition with outsiders such as the reader.

An important aspect both of the knowledge people already have and of their attitudes is that they may well perceive and rank the food problems they experience quite differently from any outside 'expert'. We need constantly to ask: does the group with whom we are concerned perceive poor diet or malnutrition as an important problem? Are they interested in attempting to change their pattern of food consumption, or do they have other problems which in their view are more pressing? Or do they, perhaps, view themselves as people whose problems cannot be tackled at all? Do they find the act of conceptualising aspects of their lives as 'problems' to which there might be 'solutions', both difficult and unfamiliar?

Conventional assessments have also fostered a negative view of traditional food customs. To take one example, it may be reported, quite correctly, that in Chinese tradition a woman who has just given birth is advised to avoid beef, mutton, and certain fish, as well as some vegetables (watercress and radishes) (Wheeler and Tan, 1983). This gives the impression that the woman's diet might be limited and even deficient. What also needs to be said is that the woman is encouraged to eat chicken, pork, offals, eggs, a large number of other vegetables, and some specially prepared 'nourishing dishes', as well as the staple foods (rice and noodles). The boundaries of acceptable food choice are well defined, but are not likely to lead to a highly restricted diet *per se,* unless some other constraints such as those associated with poverty or isolation are also operating.

In all cultures, there are foods which may not be eaten either at all, or only at certain times, times and places at which eating is inappropriate, and methods of handling food which are unacceptable. The precise content of these rules varies but the existence of rules is universal. It is also universal that within these negative, or proscriptive boundaries, the range of food choice is very wide indeed. Within them, there is scope for attitudes that relate to personal preferences, ideas about status and prestige in relation to food, and patterns of eating peculiar to particular households. However, for most of the 'ultra-poor', *practicality* excludes the luxury of making the choices these attitudes imply. For some of them, there may be one cheap dish – a ragi porridge, perhaps – which has to be eaten day in, day out, with almost no variety.

Change in food choice

It is against this background that we consider the potential for nutrition education. There is certainly no doubt that food choices can be influenced from outside the family and its immediate social setting. Were it not so, no advertising agency would be employed by a food manufacturer. Indeed, advertising ought to be understood as one form of nutrition education. If increased agricultural production is regarded as more important than distributional issues then the purpose of nutrition education could be confined to the act of promoting wider acceptance of the food crops and varieties best suited to the pattern of production to which they are committed.

The experience of advertisers is that purchasers can be persuaded to try new foods, or new versions of familiar foods, or simply old foods in new packages. The success of Coca-Cola and yeast bread in tropical countries, and of pasta foods from southern Europe in Britain, are examples of this. It is noteworthy that advertisements are designed almost exclusively to address 'attitude', and to associate status and success, or comfort and love, with a certain food. Some advertisements address 'knowledge', but with a strong emphasis on 'attitude' and prestige as well: the implication is, 'this knowledge will make you a better parent'.

The most successfully advertised foods are generally those which offer some advantage rather than simply presenting a novelty. Bread is an easily handled 'takeaway' food which succeeds in urban, mobile societies where food snacks need to be quick and portable. For the middle- and upper-class woman, processed baby milks offer the advantage of freedom from the immediate demands of a baby – they offer freedom to work and socialise, while at the same time giving a conspicuous indication of the care being lavished on the child. Success by advertisers and manufacturers in changing food behaviour involves careful study of what people want, and of ways in which new food products relate to their attitudes and sense of status.

But of course, advertising is not the only reason for change in food choice. More often, perhaps, changes are a response to alterations in the price and availability of different foods. These may simply reflect the vagaries of weather and the behaviour of markets, but may also be due to the efforts of business organisations or of government to manipulate food choices.

Another reason for a shift in family food habits may be a change in lifestyle, such as that which may result from migration, whether to a city or another country, or where settlement or resettlement programmes are under way. Changing lifestyles may also reflect upward economic and social movement. Similarly, when a new family is established after a marriage, or when absent members rejoin a household, food behaviour can and does change. All these are times when households may be open to considering new foods, new food preparation methods, and new valuations of the social and prestige value of food and drink (Lowe, 1980; Brown, 1980).

If changes in food choice arise mainly from changes in circumstances such as these, or from changes in attitude, we may well ask what role nutrition education should play. Two approaches may be distinguished, labelled for convenience 'didactic' and 'problem-posing'. The first is typical of much nutrition and health education carried out in aid programmes and development projects. The model is essentially of a one-way transfer of information, with the objective of changing a specific aspect of behaviour. Examples might be 'breast-feed your child', or 'eat more green vegetables'. A generalised statement might be: 'do this, because I *know* that your health will be improved if you follow my informed advice'. Often the use of this technique is preceded by information-gathering about problems and practices of the recipients, but always it is the educator who makes the analysis. Often, too, it is assumed that those to whom the instructions are addressed need to learn just one simple thing at a time, and that when they have accepted this small package of knowledge and put it into practice, they can proceed to the next one.

The didactic type of nutrition education is open to a number of criticisms, some general and some operational. It assumes that the people concerned are not using resources efficiently, and are not allocating them rationally because they are 'ignorant'. Thus the educator's job is seen as to impart knowledge, and the idea that it might be possible to *exchange* information is not admitted. Yet, as we have seen, there is good reason to expect that rural people are already knowledgeable about foods and recipes relevant to their circumstances. Research is badly needed in this aspect of indigenous technical knowledge and on systems of explanation, but meanwhile, we can never safely assume that people are ignorant merely on the grounds that their feeding practices are not what we expect.

There are numerous examples of inappropriate nutrition education where it has been assumed that people need information, and where the problems of 'practicality' are not taken into account. Women of the Ga tribe in West Africa have been taught about child feeding when their practices were already good. Very poor women in Bombay have been told to use more green vegetables despite the impossibly high prices they would have to pay for them. In many such instances, educators pre-judge the situation by using materials from standard syllabuses without thinking about whether people need the advice they are given, or whether they can make use of it when their food choices are severely limited by low income, indebtedness, heavy work burdens, time constraints, and a rigid division of labour between the sexes. Poor families are at the bottom of a very complex structure which imposes disadvantage on them. The educator is not going to make any difference to that situation simply by giving them information.

In general, then, ignorance is not a primary bottleneck, so nutrition education in the didactic sense is rarely effective in very poor societies. It does not address real problems. There may still be some point, however, in exploring the potential for exchanging information and developing dialogue with people in need.

Problem-posing education

Many well-informed and thoughtful educators are aware of the need to offer practicable and timely information, and they do investigate what can be done in local conditions. But few indeed ask: 'What effect does this education have on attitudes, and ultimately on consumption?' And fewer still recognise that health or nutrition education may have a negative effect because of its lack of sensitivity to people's real wants and needs. In many adult education programmes there is no sign that anyone has learned from advertisers the lesson of building on a perceived need or filling a gap in demand.

Critics of didactic nutrition education have said that it is worthless, pointing to the widespread experience that people fail to learn, their children do not grow bigger, and basic problems are unaffected. Indeed, one can come to no other conclusion than that such programmes are harmful, because they support the idea that ignorance causes malnutrition, and that parents are to blame unless they learn to do better. Even where the education programme is not promoting the particular foods for which production increases are taking place, this educational approach is rooted in the same ideology – the ideology of development as something planned by experts and imposed on people.

Fortunately, however, there are examples of programmes in which nutritionists have made a more constructive contribution. In these instances, nutrition is usually part of a package offered to rural people and from which they can choose. One instance in Guatemala has been described by Praun (1982), who had first experienced the negative effects of didactic nutrition education. Reacting to this experience, she went on with colleagues to adopt an approach of the kind often described in adult education literature as 'problem-posing', 'dialogic' or 'participatory', because it involves discussion between the educator and the local people from the earliest planning stages. The model here is of a two-way transfer of information, and a general statement might be: 'Given my capabilities as a (nutrition/health/agricultural) professional, and your range of problems, what should we work on? I can give you technical and descriptive information if you can specify for me the problems to which it needs to be applied.'

In the area where Praun worked, the prevalance of malnutrition has been increasing. In 1970, some 75 per cent of children under five presented a range of defined 'malnutrition problems'; in 1980, the corresponding figure was 82 per cent. When conventional didactic programmes were organised, people commented: 'what you say is very interesting but we can't use it, we are poor' (Praun, 1982, p.31). When the 'problem-posing approach' was adopted, local groups were given an opportunity to discuss the problems they were most aware of, and the resources available to them. The difficulty was not that the people were ignorant of local resources, but that, like other deprived and oppressed groups, they despaired of ever being able 'to do something by themselves'.

The programme was initiated through discussions with representatives from a number of villagers who then returned home and sought a local decision as to whether people wished to join the programme. Those groups which did join were expected to choose two people who could commit themselves to participate in courses every ten weeks and then work in their home locality as '*promotores*' for a period of two years. Organised activity within the programme centred on the courses given to regional groups of *promotores*. Each course lasted four full days, and took place in a centre where participants, and topics such as 'the nutrition situation in our locality' were developed through a set of questions. Typical questions dealt with food prices and availability, local production, family diets, common child illnesses, and family food budgets. The participants organised themselves into small groups to gather the necessary information about each item and then to present it at a meeting of all members of the course.

Praun (1982, p.33) goes on to comment that: 'Because the programme was called "Nutrition", people expected to receive demonstrations of how to make new food preparations; so using a limited amount of money, different food items were bought at the local market.' However, not wishing to repeat the mistakes of the 'didactic' type of programme, the organisers did not demonstrate recipes, but instead asked the local members of the course to prepare a demonstration. 'It was surprising for everyone to realise how many new recipes could be obtained using local foods and the knowledge of the participants.' After some two and a half years, 61 *promotores* were participating in such courses and 'periodically' visiting a total of 281 villages, 'several of which were able to develop their own projects', including farms and gardens run by local groups, purchases of fertiliser and seed, and the organisation of day-care centres for children.

Work of this kind is associated particularly with the writings of Paolo Freire (1970, 1973), who looked on it as an essential part of the process of transforming society and social relations. His view of 'problem-posing education' was that it must involve educators and people in a reflection on their situation, and that it should lead to 'revolutionary' action for change. Others who have written about Freire's methodology do not follow him thus far. Yet it is necessary to realise that an open-ended, problem-centred approach to adult education in low-income countries almost inevitably arouses interest in social change and hence leads to political repercussions. This was the case in Praun's experience, where pressure from local landowners eventually resulted in her team's departure.

The latter outcome may be taken as a tribute to the relevance of the programme; the more conventional, didactic type of nutrition education would usually be so ineffective that no landowner could possibly have cause to object. However, there is arguably very little value in a 'relevant' programme if its premature withdrawal is enforced. That may remind one again of the conclusions of the United Nations researchers (UNRISD, 1974) who were quoted in Chapter 7: 'the organisation of working cultivators and labourers is necessary' if they are to participate and share in the benefit of production increases. Moreover, their organisation must be strong enough to counterbalance the political and economic pressures, and even the violence, that can stem from other organised interest groups. If strong organisations already exist, problem-posing education might well provide a means of exploring and extending their agendas for action. If such organisations do not exist, however, this approach may simply expose local leaders, as well as nutritionists and others involved, to harassment or worse.

Problem-posing nutrition education is not something to be introduced everywhere, therefore, but a good deal can be learned by thinking about its implications. Instead of addressing people's food choices directly, the aim is rather to open a dialogue on 'choice about choices' (Wheeler, 1982). That gives nutritionists a rather difficult role. Their place in didactic education is clear enough: they hold the knowledge which, it is assumed, the recipients need, and given some training in communication skills, they should be effective in changing behaviour. In problem-posing education, however, knowledge is kept in the background unless it is required. Working with social scientists as well as with local people, the nutritionist may be involved in discussion about social structures and village resources more than about food distribution.

Even where 'problem-posing' is not appropriate or acceptable, we can use some of these ideas and move away from didactic teaching. There are many situations, from consumer advice to in-school education, where the educator can first discuss with people what information may be relevant to the decisions they have to take rather than presenting pre-packaged facts and figures.

10 Professional roles and research*

Consumers and nutritionists

Up to the present, nutritionists have typically been employed in health education in designing feeding programmes, or as advisers on food and nutrition policy. They have been expected to measure the nutritional status of populations and monitor the nutritional qualities of foods, and give warning of toxicity problems, or point out where the fortification of staples could be of benefit.

As examples of some established roles, we can quote the work of nutritionists in helping to define criteria in crop breeding research; we can also note that they have sometimes been asked to advise on agricultural programmes where there is concern about malnutrition in the locality. In both contexts, the assumption has been that there are questions to be answered by nutritionists about the supply of food – about what food should be given to the people thought to be malnourished, and about how crop breeding could improve the supply of particular nutrients.

However, new roles have been identified in previous chapters, all of which can be described as 'problem analysis'. They include such activities as:

---

*This chapter is based on material prepared by Barbara Harriss, Adam Pain, Philip Payne, and Paul Richards. See Harriss (1982), Pain (1982), Payne (1976) and Richards (1979, 1982).

1. providing information about the distribution of malnutrition in the population;
2. elucidating the processes which give rise to malnutrition in particular kinds of environmental and socio-economic circumstances;
3. helping to assess priorities for improved nutrition as between different categories of people;
4. monitoring and evaluating trends in nutritional status.

In addition, we described in Chapter 6 how it should be possible to find a modified role for the nutritionist in agricultural projects and programmes. This is to provide evidence about what kinds of households most often contain malnourished individuals; what part those families play in the production process; to what extent their condition is the result of insecure food availability, or disease, or social discrimination; how such people would be affected by changes in the crop varieties grown; and how the nutritional effects of a development programme could be monitored and used for management decisions.

These tasks illustrate a very important point about the new approach. They suggest that for nutrition, as with all other technical subjects, the limitations of its impact on human welfare stem less from levels of competence or knowledge, than from how well we make the connection between academic professionalism and problems experienced and perceived by the majority of the population. Consequent on this, and in the context of rural society, the new approach will require nutritionists to 'interact' with and identify with rural people in a number of ways, not merely to study them, but to listen to them and be prepared to learn from them. Parallel with this are points to be made about the way in which agriculturalists may learn from the experience and knowledge of farmers.

To put these points in context, we need to remember that scientific knowledge is never as objective as it seems. The significance of scientific discoveries for policy differs according to their interests. It is an illusion to think that scientific research can come up with recommendations for food policy (or anything else) which will automatically command a consensus. It is, however, right to be sensitive to the fact that research may have a

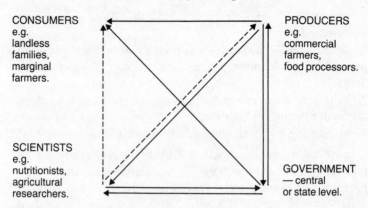

Figure 10.1   A simplified view of interactions and 'dialogue' between four of the many kinds of participant in the food system

different influence on the various interest groups. But any influence is only possible if the scientist is willing to engage in dialogue and interact in an appropriate manner with each group to explore the likely relevance of scientific findings for them.

Figure 10.1 illustrates in a highly simplified way some of the directions in which such dialogue may proceed. Bold lines indicate the well-established interaction that exists between scientists and government by virtue of the employment of nutritionists and agriculturists in administration and planning, and through public funding for research. Their dialogue is both direct and through written professional communications. Bold lines also indicate an active dialogue between producers and government. This dialogue takes the form of active lobbying by farmers' organisations on the one hand, and of signals from government through price supports, levies and taxes on the other.

The striking thing about these relationships as they commonly exist, and as Figure 10.1 illustrates them is that the consumer is rarely in a position to have his or her point of view made known. According to the conventional wisdom of the west, his or her interests are taken care of by the mechanism of 'consumer sovereignty' which is operative in 'free markets'. On entering a shop, a person is free to spend money as he or she chooses. They are not forced to buy 'nutritious' food, or 'convenience' food, or merely tasty food, but can choose; and if prices in one shop are high, they can go to another. This, however, is only the final transaction in the food system, and we saw in Chapter 8 that at many other points in the system markets are not free. Moreover, in many societies where women buy food, women who are in employment may have no choice but to pay more for a food which is quick to prepare, and may have little time to seek out shops with low prices.

The consumer sovereignty model works best in practice where there is a large number of individual consumers and where many small businesses or producers service their needs. Where large corporations are operating at the wholesale or agro-processing level, and where the larger cultivators are organised within strong farmers' associations, a more realistic picture is that developed by Keynes and Galbraith of a society composed of 'countervailing powers', that is, of large businesses and multinational corporations negotiating with powerful producers, and with the government also taking no interest in the process. In this situation, neither the bargaining power nor the 'sovereignty' of consumers and those who hire out their labour is very great. Where trade unions exist, they may increase the bargaining power of the poor in labour markets. However, there are no forceful consumer bodies in India, nor in other developing countries, and those that are active in western countries tend to represent a middle-class interest and not the poor.

Remedies for this situation are well outside the scope of the nutritionist or agriculturist, but he or she must be aware of the problem. When members of either profession are recruited into the service of a State food corporation or a multinational company, they are expected to further that organisation's interests, perhaps indirectly, perhaps in an advocacy role, by seeking and presenting evidence favourable to that organisation. Where a nutritionist has, by contrast, a degree of independence from such organisations, the question arises as to whether he or she might take an advocacy role of an opposite kind, on behalf of labourers' families, marginal farmers, or the poor in general. In 1983, Indian nutritionists did this by expressing professional concern to the Central Government about four issues: 1. the large scale replacement of coarse grains production by that of soya bean intended for export for cattle feed; 2. the increased acreage down to sugar cane, to the detriment of potato production, and large, subsidised loans to the sugar manufacturing industry; 3. the decline in per caput availability of foodgrains and pulses from 1961–81; 4. perpetuated deficiencies in iron and vitamins A and B complex (Bull. MIDS, 1983, p.564). The Government's response is unknown.

Such a nutritionist should clearly be cautious about being an uninvited advocate for causes which people have not defined for themselves. A certain amount might be done, however, in giving consumers more information about trends in food marketing, or in using 'problem-posing' education of the kind described in the previous chapter to help the poor formulate their own priorities. But little may be achieved if the people concerned do not have some bargaining power and the capability of protecting their interests.

Agricultural research

Discussion about the aims of agricultural research, and choice of topics to be investigated, is one area where we might expect to see a fruitful interaction between scientists and other interested groups. For example, if one goal is an increase in rice yield, discussion between scientists, farmers and extension staff might be useful in identifying constraints on yield which are experienced in practice. This might lead to suggestions that research should be focused on water management or perhaps pest control rather than, say, fertiliser response or plant breeding. Even if such discussions were not held, we might expect that the programme for research would be decided by reference to explicit criteria of some sort. Very probably these would be criteria relating to efficient use of research funds and facilities.

In practice, however, there is rarely evidence of any sort of systematic procedure. Choices are made with only minimal interactions between scientists and extension staff or planners, and with no evident reference to identifiable scientific criteria. We therefore need to examine other factors that may influence decisions. For example, the interests of scientists are inevitably affected by the thrust of career ambitions and publication objectives, and also by a range of more technical factors. Some of the latter are related to the current state of knowledge in biochemistry, physiology and genetics, and the possibility of applying theories or pursuing advances in these subjects at the same time as the crop is being improved.

In this context, it is significant that although plant breeding is only one aspect of agricultural research, it has dominated approaches towards raising crop yields. This is partly the result of a history of notable achievements, but also reflects a belief that this type of improvement in crop production is directly amenable to technical manipulation by the professional scientist, without need for complex multidisciplinary programmes. Problems of low yield and disease can be solved by developing new varieties, and this approach has scientific interest in its own right. In Sri Lanka, for example, breeding has raised the yield *potential* of rice from 2.4 t/ha in the 1950s to nearly 7.8 t/ha for the modern (BG) varieties. However, the national average yields have only risen from 1.7 t/ha to 3.9 t/ha over the same period. Plant breeders clearly get results, but more could arguably have been achieved by wider study of practical problems experienced by farmers.

In many countries, breeding for increased yield was initiated at a time when there was concern about large-scale food shortages. The emergence a little later of a parallel concern about widespread dietary protein deficiency led to research on improved levels of protein content in cereals. There are technical problems here of some considerable scientific interest, not least because cereals with a high protein yield tend to be characterised by low protein quality (i.e. amino acid balance) as Table 10.1 shows. However, solutions are now chiefly of academic interest as far as human problems are concerned since neither lack of protein nor low protein quality is currently thought to be a major cause of malnutrition.

Among the studies which contributed to this change of view,

Table 10.1   *Estimates of the protein content of cereals utilisable by children (For an explanation of protein quality, see page 77 above; total protein–energy ratio may be taken as a measure of 'yield' in this context.)*

Cereals and sources of data	Total protein/ energy ratio (column 1)	Quality as efficiency of utilisation (%) (column 2)	Utilisable protein content (%) (column 1) × (column 2)
Maize			
Tasker *et al.*1962	0.13	36	4.8
Opaque–2 hybrid, Bressani 1966;			
Payne 1976		60 – 70	6 – 7
Millet			
Kurien *et al.* 1961	0.12	43	5.3
Rice			
Joseph *et al.* 1963	0.073	66	4.8
Tasker *et al.* 1962	0.097	63	6.1
Wheat			
Penemangalore *et al.* 1962	0.11	49	5.2

Source: After Payne (1976).

there were several in which children (usually in orphanages) were fed carefully standardised diets in controlled amounts. For example, Pereira *et al.* (1973) gave children a rice-based diet containing very small amounts of legume and other vegetables, simulating the food normally consumed in local villages. When fed in amounts corresponding to the recommended level of energy intake for that age group, the children achieved 'standard' growth rates. However, the village children grew more slowly; they were given the same type of diet in their own homes, but were found to have eaten much smaller quantities. The diet of both groups was then supplemented with lysine. In neither case was any growth improvement found. Pereira interpreted these results as showing that the protein requirements of the orphanage children were fully met by the cereal diet. The growth of the village children, on the other hand, was limited by their relatively low energy intake, so that again, no response to lysine could be expected. Their diet might be judged inadequate, but not because the percentage of lysine was low.

The efficiency of utilisation of protein from cereals is limited by the balance of amino acids in the cereals. But provided sufficient cereal is consumed to meet energy and total protein needs, as it was with Pereira's orphanage children, then conventional varieties nearly always contain enough lysine and the other amino acids to meet requirements, even of preschool children. Plant breeders have produced high-lysine strains of maize, one of which, known as 'opaque-2', is likely to have a utilisable protein content of between 6 and 7 per cent, as compared with about 4.8 per cent for other maize varieties. Even the lower figure for maize, however, and the equally low figures for rice (Table 10.1), represent an adequate intake for a child who is consuming enough of the cereal to supply his or her energy needs.

One might think that the publication of such findings (Ryan *et al.*, 1974; Payne, 1976) would by now have diverted plant breeders away from the goal of developing high-protein varieties. Yet considerable time and effort has continued to be spent in examining various strategies for raising protein levels in individual species or improving protein quality. An 'inbuilt momentum' within the research is evident which needs to be understood in terms of at least two facets of research activity – scientific and institutional.

On the scientific level, it can seem that agendas for research are partly based on technical interest and partly on the relative ease with which problems can be tackled. Yield improvement has tended to be the first aim of the breeders because it is fairly easy to achieve results. Improving protein quality and content is much more difficult, but for that reason may be perceived as more challenging, and therefore it may be placed high on the intellectual agenda as a subject having interest in its own right.

Plant breeders work by using a range of techniques for combining desirable or superior forms of a particular characteristic into one plant variety. Yield is one such characteristic, determined by many physiological functions within the plant, and its genetic base is quite complex. Yet it is easy to deal with because a high-yielding variety can be identified simply by going into the field and weighing its yield. The scientists' expression, 'breeding for yield', implies that attributes from different varieties are carefully brought together into a particular configuration that will predictably produce a high-yielding variety. This is very far from the case, and what has happened, almost without exception, is that higher yielding varieties have been selected by empirical methods from crosses of parents with desirable traits. By contrast, selection for protein quality is dependent upon the use of analytical techniques for assay. Such techniques are becoming increasingly sophisticated in the pursuit of accuracy and precision, and, as a result, they are getting more time-consuming and expensive.

This, perhaps, is a clue to some of the institutional reasons for the momentum in protein-maximisation programmes. An investment in equipment and staff is necessary which may not be easily adaptable to other programmes, and some research stations therefore maintain their commitment to a protein programme. It is noteworthy, however, that improved protein content in rice is not felt to be justified as a research priority by the International Rice Research Institute (IRRI), because of the urgency of other problems such as pest resistance and tolerance to various environmental conditions (Nanda and Coffman, 1979; IRRI, 1982). Rice has a good amino acid balance, though a limited protein content (Table 10.1), so there is little point in seeking to raise the proportion of lysine as was done with maize.

It is also significant that, despite concern about protein, breeding programmes in many countries have focused on cereals rather than legumes, until very recently. This is ostensibly because cereals feature more prominently in the diet of the world's population. They contribute about 70 per cent, and legumes only 20 per cent of world supplies of plant protein (Jalil and Tahir, 1973). But the focus of breeding programmes also reflects the profit margins associated with cereal growing in developed countries, and the business interests involved in promoting wheat (or to a lesser extent, maize and rice). Only soya among the legumes is backed by a comparable lobby.

Protein content in grain legumes is, of course, already quite high (20-45 per cent) and it is difficult to account for some current projects which aim to breed for even higher protein levels. Yields are notoriously poor for many legume species, and there are unresolved pest control problems. These would seem to be more urgent priorities for research, especially in India, where they are a factor in the declining per caput production of pulses. Legume research, indeed, is one of several topics which might be approached differently if scientists were more aware of the processes which generate poverty and malnutrition. Instead of asking: 'what is the protein content of this crop?', they might be more willing to ask: 'what is the effect on livelihoods of the relative decline of pulses?' Research might then be directed to making the cultivation of pulses more worthwhile for the marginal farmer.

Divergent goals and hidden agendas

With the emphasis of so much agricultural research and planning on *production*, those individuals who feel that agriculture ought also to be concerned with nutritional welfare or with creating jobs are apt to experience a discontinuity between their values and this narrowly defined economic purpose. In commenting on that discontinuity, United Nations researchers have argued that policies should be formulated around 'improved family liveli-hood rather than around production targets' (see page 159 above).

In agricultural research, there is an additional conflict of purpose arising from the high valuation which is placed on activities having scientific or technical interest in their own right, such as plant breeding and work on protein quality. Agricultural research may thus be pulled three ways by divergent sets of values – firstly, those focused on economics and production; then those based on livelihoods; and thirdly, those aimed at 'technically sweet' innovation. This is not surprising, since

210   *Food and Nutrition Policy and Agriculture*

similarly divergent value systems are found to influence other branches of technology (Pacey, 1983, p.102). Industrial research, for example, may also be subject to conflicts between economic goals and aims which reflect scientific interests (Galbraith, 1972, chapter 15). Moreover, goals reflecting consumer interests or social needs often prove to be surprisingly incompatible with both economic goals and scientific interests.

Neglect of priorities based on a consideration of consumer or social needs is demonstrated for agricultural research in a literature review by Biggs (1981). He notes that analytical tools exist for establishing development-oriented priorities where there are conflicts between production, employment, income distribution and similar goals. However, it does not seem that these tools are used at all, whether it be in international, national or local research institutions. Furthermore, a study of American agricultural scientists has shown that research goals related to health and nutrition are regarded as 'not intrinsically important' (Busch *et al.*, 1980, p.10).

National and international bodies responsible for formulating agricultural research policies frequently mention nutritional and social priorities, but significantly, they never confront the value systems which prevent these priorities being taken seriously. In America, one such review of policies having a worldwide perspective has come from the Commission on International Relations of the National Research Council (NRC, 1977). It is clear from their list of priorities that yet again the problems of world nutrition are conceived of as stemming from insufficient *production*, and questions of land ownership or of entitlement to food are ignored. In view of the points made in previous chapters, we would expect policy reviews of this kind to specify that new agricultural technologies for production, storage and processing should raise productivity per unit of capital and per unit of land without causing a net decrease in employment. Therein, of course, lies the real challenge of innovation, because the trend has always been for technological development to increase productivity per unit of labour whatever happens to land and to capital. But this challenge is evaded by the American Commission, and they are left with the seeds of a contradiction.

The more productive technologies they advocate could lead to unemployment and so reduce effective demand, which they also say they want to raise.

To a striking degree, the research priorities for agriculture in India set out in the sixth five-year plan echo these American proposals (Government of India, 1981). Again production is emphasised, with plant breeding aimed at yield improvement. The main difference is the stress laid on energy conservation; there are also differences in the crops to which special attention is to be paid – oilseeds, pulses, vegetables and tree crops.

The most influential of the international bodies is probably the Consultative Group on International Agricultural Research (CGIAR), an offshoot of the World Food Council responsible for the thirteen major international research centres. Each international centre is concerned with specific agro-ecological regions, and specific food crops or animals. We have already referred to IRRI's work on rice, located in the Philippines. CIMMYT does research on wheat, barley, triticale and maize, and is located in Mexico; it justifies breeding for high quality protein not merely for the possible relevance to human diets, but also with better animal nutrition in view (CGIAR, 1980). ICRISAT, outside Hyderabad, aims at genetic improvement of sorghum and millet, chickpea, pigeon pea and groundnut, and at developing 'principles for farming systems which will be applicable over a wide range of dryland environments' (CGIAR, 1980, p.4).

One irony in most of the formal statements of policy issued by national or international bodies is that the priorities they establish do not readily filter through to the agricultural scientists. As early as 1974, it was shown at ICRISAT that energy content rather than protein ought to be maximised in the cereals of the semi-arid tropics (Ryan *et al.*, 1974), but that did not halt the momentum of work elsewhere aimed at raising protein yields. This underlines the point made earlier that research seems unrelated to explicit, identifiable criteria in many instances. Reasons for this are connected with the organisation of research – its administration and division of labour. The personnel involved are likely, after all, to behave like members of other bureaucracies and seek first and foremost to secure their own interests, namely, perpetuation and expansion of the work, prestige for the institution, and operation of a satisfactory career structure.

In this respect, Schaffer's views on the nature of public policy in general offer many insights. He suggests that formal policy documents do not have meaning as statements of intention. Organisations have goals and programmes of a deep-seated, unacknowledged kind which constitute their 'hidden agendas'. Policies are envisaged by Schaffer as emerging from these agendas through a defensive operation which enables policy-makers to remain unaware of unacknowledged goals concerning the survival of the organisation, which thus remain truly hidden, even from those who apparently set the agendas. The formal programme which is then produced depends on the extent to which statistical and scientific information can be assembled to demonstrate the necessity of activities which are felt to be important. No conscious deception is involved, but assumptions are made in assembling such data that have the effect of disguising subjective judgement as objective fact. This pre-empts debate about the decisions concerned, and allows members of the organisation to believe that their interest in expansion and prestige is compatible with their social concern about what the statistics reveal (Schaffer and Lamb, 1981).

In this context, it is worth noticing that the actual role of much agricultural research in developing countries has been to facilitate the transfer of technologies developed in Europe and North America. This in itself may tell us something about the hidden agendas of the research organisations and the context in which their members view career advancement. As Chambers (1983, p186) points out, the researcher who works on biological nitrogen fixation may ultimately help small farmers, but if he works on crop responses to chemical nitrogen, he helps only farmers who can afford to buy fertiliser. However, successful work on the chemical option is more likely to attract financial support, not least from fertiliser companies, and so may lead to new opportunities for the researcher to advance his work.

Research on chemical fertiliser and other components of

production packages from developed countries strengthens the position of commercial agriculture and of 'proto-capitalist' farmers with investible surplus (Byres, 1981). This will be seen as an advantage in certain quarters; it may indeed be that support for capitalist farming and avoidance thereby of land reform is part of the 'hidden agenda' of some research, as it is alleged to be of the American interests which have pushed HYV packages (George, 1977, p.125)

Linear versus interactive research

Although agendas for agricultural research may be largely unacknowledged in written policy statements, they are in some ways clearly expressed in the buildings and physical terrain of the research stations themselves, in their methods of administration, and in their means of accountability. All these things are arranged, though not deliberately, in ways that tend to exclude from the research process the intended beneficiaries: that is, the farmers. Yields achieved by the latter in their own fields, however good, are discounted. Innovations made by farmers, and processing technologies developed 'off-station', tend to be disregarded. In the past the wheel has tended to be reinvented inside the barbed-wire perimeter fence (Richards, 1981).

Learning from farmers could be the biggest improvement in research that is feasible within the present political economy. More radical departures from existing procedures would require considerable decentralisation of responsibility, and there is to date no constituency for this. However, learning from farmers may itself depend on some loosening of bureaucratic commitments and changes in professional attitudes and practice. Where specialists identify themselves with a recognised profession, they often discourage new ideas if these are inconsistent with their view of a professional role. The tendency is for such people to see their vocation as a 'closed system' – a body of 'self-sufficient knowledge and technique'. In one study of professionals in the public health field, it was noted that this sense of self-sufficiency led most of them to regard consultation with lay people as 'either unnecessary or potentially harmful', even where those people's interests were at issue (Sewell, 1977).

With regard to nutrition research, we have made two examinations of the literature, one restricted to 1978–9 (Wheeler, 1982), the other focusing on papers relevant to India (Cutler, 1982a). In both studies, we noted the persistence of some well-established lines of research. There was a preponderance of papers on malnutrition in children, and on anthropometry, but apart from that, research continued to be much more concerned with the properties and use of foods than with the nutritional problems of populations as perceived by themselves.

The tendency for particular kinds of research (and technological innovation) to persist over long periods by a continuous extrapolation of established ideas is another result of the professionals' closed system. It tends to produce a *linear* pattern of innovation (Pacey, 1983), in contrast to the more informal *interactive* mode of research and development which is possible when applied scientists are willing to learn from farmers (or housewives, or artisans). Links with the 'problem-posing' approach to education discussed in the previous chapter (p.195) should be apparent.

Farm level grain storage provides examples of both approaches. Extrapolation of conventional engineering and scientific experience has led to a range of designs for concrete silos and metal bins. But one British research institute which used this approach discovered during field trials in Africa that its silos were too costly and had minor technical faults. Slowly the researchers recognised that indigenous structures of mud-wall construction had very real advantages. After that, the work became much more 'interactive', and led in one instance to publication of a manual on detailed improvements to traditional grain stores (Malawi Ministry of Agriculture, 1973).

Similarly, 'experts' visiting Andhra Pradesh recommended a range of metal grain bins on the basis of conventional engineering criteria. This was again a 'linear' study, extrapolating western technical experience, and as Greeley points out, the 'experts' made no measurements of local storage losses, nor did they study the 'operational feasibility' or socio-economic impact of their metal bins. Implicit in this approach 'was a belief that traditional farm-level storage practices were incapable of improvement' (Greeley, 1978, p.43).

Work on storage in Andhra Pradesh was later taken up by an interdisciplinary group using quite different and markedly more 'interactive' methods. Their starting point was a study of grain losses from traditional storage containers. These were less than expected – about 5 per cent of the grain stored – and showed the worth of the traditional techniques. Minor improvements in existing types of container were then devised, some of which eliminated all sources of loss. A professional engineer helped develop the modifications, but they were 'finalised in consultation with village masons and farmers' (Greeley, 1978, p.49). After that, the improvements depended for their implementation on the skills of local artisans, so there was a gain for rural livelihoods.

One practical reason why interactive research ought to be stressed is that it can help to ensure that innovation is relevant to local resources and needs. According to UNRISD (1974), it is relevant to seed testing in local conditions, to studies of husbandry methods, and to work on water management. On all these topics, a continuing dialogue between farmers and researchers is possible, with extension staff also involved. Indeed, the extensionist can and should be something of an expert on traditional agriculture, local geography and local social values, and so may be especially well placed to interpret farmers' ideas to the scientists.

Another good example of interactive research concerns the variegated grasshopper, a pest which damages cassava crops in the forest zone of West Africa (Richards, 1979). This insect is not easily dealt with by high technology methods such as aerial spraying. Thus after several bad outbreaks in southern Nigeria during 1965-70, a research team set out to examine other possibilities. They quickly found that farmers saw the insect almost daily, had observed its life cycle accurately, and had experimented with control strategies. One or two farmers even anticipated and so helped to confirm the control techniques which the research team ultimately recommended, namely digging up egg-laying sites.

Other instances have been documented where it has been possible to learn from farmers about soils, plant species, and other environmental features (Howes, 1979). Chapman (1974, 1982) has shown that the folklore of farmers in Bihar contains a vast wealth of knowledge about weather and planting dates, and Benneh (1970) points out that professionals waste time when they do expensive research on what farmers already know. Biggs mentions an instance where priorities in a research station were significantly altered in the light of what was learned from farmers about yields of triticale (Biggs, 1982). This was yet another case where interactive research really did work, and further practical instances have been reported from Central America (Hildebrand, 1981) and Africa (Collinson, 1981). So interactive research cannot be dismissed as an utopian ideal.

However, the decision to opt for an interactive rather than a 'high technology' programme can raise some awkward questions about who is to participate. What people in Nigeria know about grasshoppers depends very much on their particular interests. Some who use the insects as food distinguish the different species very precisely. Farmers who grow yams may associate them with other pests that attack this crop. And during the research work cited, some women in eastern Nigeria refused to say what they knew because they earned money preparing variegated grasshoppers for sale as food, and were understandably suspicious of a programme which aimed to reduce the availability of their raw material.

We should appreciate that it is not only among farmers and village people that knowledge depends on group interests. Scientists can be unaware of the 'hidden' agendas influencing their research choices because of what they take for granted, or because judgements based on interest seem to them 'purely technical'. But the decision-making process is underminded when 'political', that is interest-based considerations are disguised as, or confused with technical considerations. Consequently, discovering and spelling out the relationships between knowledge and interests is an important analytical obligation for all groups involved in research (Richards, 1982).

Conclusion

If an interactive mode of research were to develop in the direction of better collaboration between people in different disciplines as well as collaboration with farmers, it could lead to agriculturalists becoming more responsive to suggestions about nutritional priorities for research. What would these be? In place of the existing interest in breeding for protein yield, there could be much greater interest in foods that provide energy at the lowest possible cost – the coarse grains, and cassava. Further, UNRISD (1974, p.54) argues that 'special attention should be given to holding down input costs' for farmers, and suggests how research on drought and pest resistant crop varieties on inter-cropping and organic manures might be relevant. The ultimate objective would be to help 'the working cultivator' for whom the high-cost inputs of green revolution technology have been a major handicap. But the same kinds of innovation would also assist in keeping the unit cost of food energy low for cultivators' families, and for many others.

If nutritionists as well as agriculturalists took a wider, more 'interactive' view of their professional roles, they could well foster greater interest in the epidemiology of malnutrition and all its social and environmental ramifications. That interest in turn could lead to a concern with the 'political economy' of food – that is, to a study of the processes which ensure that some groups of people have plenty while others do not have enough.

All this would make for a more rational, more innovative style of professional activity, but it would achieve little more if the context were one of unresponsive, ineffective or contradictory public policy. For example, we have noted a preoccupation in many countries with food production (rather than consumption), observing that during the 'green revolution', this led to 'the dissolution of rural livelihoods' (UNRISD, 1974). We could justifiably comment that to concentrate on food production is to have only half a policy; the missing half would be a policy on employment and on food entitlement, aimed at protecting and enhancing livelihoods.

Public policy for nutrition has often included the provision of supplementary foods to mothers and children. But we have already pointed out that this too is only half a policy. Measures are also required to prevent the erosion of livelihoods by interlocked food and labour markets. Progress is thus needed on two fronts simultaneously, and while on one, government agencies may properly give extra food to mothers and infants, on the other front, they must reduce the distortions in markets which trap many of the ultra-poor in their depressed positions. If the policies which provide the extra food also have the effect of increasing market distortions, they may well be self-defeating – as are the policies which promote production by means that reduce employment.

The constructive possibility which arises from recent efforts to identify 'ultra-poor' and malnourished groups more precisely is that it should be easier to design programmes that avoid these contradictions. Thus if Harriss is right in suggesting that many of the problems of the poor arise from their dependence on imperfectly functioning markets, it might make sense to by-pass these markets altogether with fair price shops and/or the distribution of welfare food.

The context of these suggestions is, of course, one in which the countervailing powers of farmers' organisations, banks and bureaucratic corporations contend to influence policy. The politician and the professional probably view this situation in different ways. The politician, should she or he feel concern about poverty, will be brought back constantly to the lack of organisation and of bargaining power among the rural poor. She or he may well regret that those poor in resources are those powerless in political leverage, because that limits what can be done. The importance of the UNRISD analysis which we have repeatedly quoted is that it goes a long way towards recognising this, and makes suggestions about two types of 'grass roots' organisation which might be deliberately encouraged. Firstly, there could be associations of small cultivators, each one covering several villages in order 'to free itself from the...large farmer domination which is suffered by village cooperatives'. Then, secondly, there could be 'mutual aid groups' for landless families, which might be fostered as micro-cooperatives, and as 'the primary unit of development for the marginalised rural sectors' (UNRISD, 1974, p.51).

These proposals might at first sight seem consistent with a liberal political ethos, but they involve a contradiction. For government to give genuine encouragement and real power (e.g. over credit) to groups of landless and poor people, it would have to by-pass many existing structures, including the state bureaucracies over which it presides.

The nutritionist has to address him or herself as a professional to the room for manoeuvre in the existing political and economic system. He or she has to devise interventions in the agricultural economy which match the needs of the malnourished and which are also feasible, in the sense that they can be steered through the tangle of countervailing interests without too much distortion, and can actually reach the malnourished.

It is with this latter point in mind that the suggestion was made about welfare feeding being more effective than attempts to modify markets. Welfare is manipulated and misused, just as market interventions are. However, if food interventions are untargeted or minimally targeted, with fewer vested interests involved, there is less likelihood of unacceptable political friction, and a better chance that those who are intended to benefit from the food provided really will. Similarly, our suggestions about agricultural research on crops that provide low-cost food energy would seem to have some feasibility. In addition, interactive research involving farmers ought also to be politically feasible in countries such as India. However, the discussion of problem-posing education in Chapter 9 illustrates the kind of tight-rope that must often be walked. Interactive research, or work on the needs of marginal farmers, may be restricted by pressures favouring production-oriented research, and by the attitudes of those who finance such studies or publish the results. The problem, which has historically defied solution in some socialist states as well as many capitalist states in the 'Third World' is to devise policy strategies which really do steer a path through contending interests and truly benefit the hungry.

Bibliography

Books and articles especially recommended for further reading are marked by an asterisk (*)

Abdulah, M. and Wheeler, E.F., *American Journal of Clinical Nutrition*, **41** no.6 (1985)

*Alleyne, G.A.O., Hay, R.W., Picou, D.I., Stanfield, J.P. and Whitehead, R.G. *Protein energy malnutrition*, London: Edward Arnold, 1977

Ashworth, A., 'Growth rates in children recovering from protein-calorie malnutrition', *British Journal of Nutrition*, **23** (1969), pp. 835–45

Ashworth, A., 'Progress in the treatment of protein-energy malnutrition', *Proceedings of the Nutrition Society*, **38** (1979), pp. 89–97

Bairagi, R., 'On best cutoff point for nutritional monitoring', *American Journal of Clinical Nutrition*, **35** (1982), pp. 769–70

Baker, D., *Indian Rural Economy, 1880–1955*, Delhi: Oxford University Press, 1983

Balaji, M. and Ramachandran, V.K., 'A report on the implication of the Food for Work Programme and the Employment Guarantee System in Ramanathapuram and Dharmapuri Districts', MIDS, Madras, mimeo, 1980

Bardhan, P.K., 'On the minimum level of living and the rural poor', *Indian Economic Review*, **5** (1) (1970a), pp.129–36

Bardhan, P.K., 'The green revolution and agricultural labourers: a correction', *Economic and Political Weekly*, **5** (46) (November 1970b), pp. 1861–2

Baster, N., 'Social indicators and social statistics', Document ESS/MISC/78–5, Rome: FAO, 1978

Bauer, R.A. (ed.), *Social Indicators*, Cambridge, Mass.: MIT Press, 1966

Bayliss-Smith, T., 'Seasonal energy relationships and food', in R. Chambers, R. Longhurst and A. Pacey (eds.), *Seasonal Dimensions to Rural Poverty*, London: Frances Pinter, 1981

Beaton, G.H. and Bengoa, J.M. (eds.), *Nutrition in Preventive Medicine*, World Health Organisation Monograph Series, no.62, Geneva, 1976

Beaton, G.H. and Ghassemi, H., 'Supplementary feeding programmes for young children in developing countries', Report prepared for UNICEF and the ACC Subcommitee on Nutrition of the UN, New York, United Nations, mimeo, 1979

Beattie, J. and Herbert, P.H., 'Estimation of the metabolic rate in the starvation state; Basal metabolism during recovery from severe malnutrition', *British Journal of Nutrition*, **1** (1947), pp.185-201

Beattie, J., Herbert, P.H. and Bell, D.J., 'Nitrogen balance during recovery from severe malnutrition', *British Journal of Nutrition*, **1** (1947), pp. 202–19

Benedict, F.G., *A Study of Prolonged Fasting*, Washington DC: Carnegie Institute, 1915

Benedict, F.G., *Human Vitality and Efficiency under a Prolonged Restricted Diet*, Washington DC: Carnegie Institute, 1919

Benneh, G., 'Technology should seek tradition', *Ceres: FAO Review*, **3** (5) (September/October 1970)

*Berg, A., *The Nutrition Factor*, Washington DC: Brookings Institute, 1973

Berkman, J.M., 'Anorexia, inanition and low basal metabolic rate', *American Journal of the Medical Sciences*, **180** (1930), pp. 411–24

Bhalla, S., 'Real wage rates of agricultural labourers in Punjab, 1961–77', *Economic and Political Weekly*, **14** (1979), no.26

*Bhatia, B.M., *Famine in India,* London: Asia Publishing House, 1963

Biggs, S.D., 'Agricultural Research: a review of social science analysis', Report to the International Development Research Centre, Ottawa, Canada (draft mimeo), 1981

Biggs, S.D., 'Generating agricultural technology: triticale for the Himalayan Hills', *Food Policy,* **7** (1982), pp. 69–82

*Binswanger, H.P. and Ryan, J.G. 'Efficiency and equity issues in *ex ante* allocation of research resources', *Indian Journal of Agricultural Economics,* **32** (1977), pp. 217–31

Blalock, H.M., *Social Statistics* (2nd edn), New York: McGraw Hill, 1979

Blaxter, K.L., *The Energy Metabolism of Ruminants* (2nd edn), London: Hutchinson, 1967

Bleiberg, F.M., Brun, T.A., Goiham, S. and Gouba, E., 'Duration of activities and energy expenditure of female farmers in dry and rainy seasons in Upper Volta', *British Journal of Nutrition,* **43** (1980), pp. 71–81

BMA, *Report of the Committee on Nutrition*, London: British Medical Association, 1950

Bradley, D.J., 'Seasonal variables in infective disease', in R. Chambers, R. Longhurst and A. Pacey, (eds.), *Seasonal Dimensions to Rural Poverty,* London: Frances Pinter, 1981

Bressani, R., in E.T. Martz and O.E. Nelson (eds.), *Proceedings of the High Lysine Corn Conference*, Washington DC: Corn Industries Research Foundation, 1966

Bressani, R., Wilson, D.L., Behar, M. and Scrimshaw, N.S., *Journal of Nutrition,* **70** (1960), p.179

Briscoe, J., 'The quantitative effect of infection on the use of food by young children in poor countries', *American Journal of Clinical Nutrition,* **32** (3) (1979), pp. 648–76

Brody, S., *Bioenergetics and Growth*, New York: Reinhold, 1945

Brown, N., 'Some observations on family eating patterns', in M. Turner (ed.), *Nutrition and Lifestyles,* London: Applied Science Publishers, 1980

Brown, R.E., 'Decreased brain weight in malnutrition', *East*

African Medical Journal, **42** (1965), pp. 584–8

Brun, T., Bleiberg, P. and Goihman, S., 'Energy expenditure of male farmers in dry and rainy seasons in Upper Volta', *British Journal of Nutrition,* **45** (1981), pp. 67–75

Bulletin, Madras Seminar Series, **13** no.11 (1983)

Burk, M.C. and Pao, E.M., 'Methodology for large-scale surveys of household and individual diets', USDA Agricultural Research Service, Home Economics Research Report, no.40, Washington, DC: USDA, 1976

Burk, M.C. and Pao, E.M., 'Analysis of food consumption survey data for developing countries', Food and Nutrition Paper, no. 16. Rome: FAO, 1980

Burnett, J., *Plenty and Want: a Social History of Diet in England,* (revised edn), London: Scholar Press, 1979

Busch, L., Lacy, W.B. and Sachs, D., 'Research policy in the agricultural sciences', Research Series 66, Department of Sociology, University of Kentucky, 1980

Byres, T.J., 'Industrialization, the peasantry and the economic debate in post-independence India', in A.V. Bhulashkar (ed.), *Towards the Socialist Transformation of the Indian Economy,* Bombay, 1972, pp.223–47

Byres, T.J., 'Land reform, industrialisation and the marketed surplus in India', in D. Lehmann (ed.), *Agrarian Reform and Agrarian Reformism,* London: Faber, 1974

*Byres, T.J., 'The new technology, class formation and class action in the Indian countryside', *Journal of Peasant Studies,* **8** (1981), pp. 405–53

Calvert, H., *Wealth and Welfare in Punjab,* (2nd edn), Lahore: Civil Gazette, 1936

Cassen, R., *India: Population, Economy, Society,* London and Basingstoke: Macmillan, 1980

CGIAR, *Report of the Consultative Group on International Agricultural Research,* Rome: World Food Council, 1980

*Chambers, R., *Rural Development: Putting the Last First,* Harlow (England): Longman, 1983

*Chambers, R., Longhurst, R. and Pacey, A., *Seasonal Dimensions to Rural Poverty,* London: Frances Pinter, 1981

Chambers, R. and Maxwell, S., 'Practical implications: the role of public works', in R. Chambers, R. Longhurst and A. Pacey (eds.), *Seasonal Dimensions to Rural Poverty*, London: Frances Pinter, 1981

Champakam, S., Srikantia, S.G. and Gopalan, R., 'Kwashiorkor and mental development', *American Journal of Clinical Nutrition*, **21** (1968), pp. 844–52

Chapman, G.P., 'Perception and regulation: a case study of farmers in Bihar', *Transactions, the Institute of British Geographers*, no. 62 (1974), pp. 71–91

Chapman, G.P., 'The folklore of the perceived environment in Bihar', Paper presented at UNICEF/FAO/NPU/ICAR Workshop on Nutrition in Agriculture, Hissar, 1982

Chapman, G.P. and Dowter, E.A., *The Green Revolution Game*, Cambridge: Marginal Context Ltd, 1982

Chaudhuri, K.N., 'Markets and traders in India during the 17th and 18th centuries', in K.N. Chaudhuri and C.J. Dewey (eds.), *Economy and Society: Essays in Indian Economic and Social History*, Delhi: Oxford University Press, 1979

Chawla, P., 'Food Corporation of India: a white elephant', *India Today*, (June 1978), pp. 32–9

*Chen, L.C., Chowdhury, A.K.M. and Huffman, S.L., 'Anthropometric assessment of energy- protein malnutrition and subsequent risk of mortality among pre-school-aged children', *American Journal of Clinical Nutrition*, **33** (1980), pp. 1836–45

Chen, L.C., Chowdhury, A.K.M. and Huffman, S.L., 'Letters to the editor', *American Journal of Clinical Nutrition* **34** (1980), pp. 2591–9

Chen, L.C., Chowdhury, A.K.M. and Huffman, S.L., 'The use of anthropometry for nutritional surveillance', *American Journal of Clinical Nutrition*, **34** (1981a), pp. 2596–9

Chen, L.C., Huq, E. and D'Souza, S., 'Sex bias in the family allocation of food and health care in rural Bangladesh', *Population and Development Review*, **7** (1981b), p. 55

Chen, L.C., Huq, E. and Huffman, S., 'A prospective study of the risk of diarrhoeal diseases according to the nutritional status of children', *American Journal of Epidemiology,* **114** no.2 (1981c), pp. 284–92

Chinnappa, B.N. and Silva, W.P.T., 'Impact of the cultivation of high-yielding varieties of paddy', in B.H. Farmer (ed.), *Green Revolution?*, London and Basingstoke: Macmillan, 1977

Chittenden, R.H., *Physiological Economy in Nutrition,* London: Heinemann, 1904

Chowdhury, A.K.M., Huffman, S.L. and Chen, L.C., 'Agriculture and nutrition in Matlab Thana, Bangladesh', in R. Chambers, R. Longhurst and A. Pacey (eds.), *Seasonal Dimensions to Rural Poverty,* London: Frances Pinter, 1981

Church, M.A., 'The importance of food consistency in supplementary feeding and the weaning process', in R. Korte (ed.), *Nutrition in Developing Countries,* Eschborn: GTZ, 1977

Church, M.A. and Doughty, J., 'The value of traditional recipes in nutrition education', *Journal of Human Nutrition,* **30** (1975), pp. 9–12

Collinson, M., 'A low cost approach to understanding farmers', *Agricultural Administration,* **8** (6) (1981), pp. 433–50

Conlin, S. and Falk, A., *Kosi Hill Area Rural Development Programme: a Study of the Socio-economy,* (2 vols.), KHARDEP Report no.3, Surbiton (England): Land Resources Development Centre, 1979

Cravioto, J., DeLicardie, E.R. and Birch, H.G., 'Nutrition, growth and neuro-integrative development', *Pediatrics,* **38** suppl. (1968), pp.319–72

Cravioto, J. and Robles, B., 'Evolution of adaptive and motor behaviour during rehabilitation from kwashiorkor', *American Journal of Orthopaedics,* **35** (1965), pp. 319–72

Culyer, A.J., Lavers, R.J. and Williams, A., 'Social indicators: health', *Social Trends,* no.2)71), pp. 31–42, London: Central Statistical Office/HMSO

Cunningham Rundles, S., 'Effects of nutritional status on immunological function', *American Journal of Clinical Nutrition,* **35** (1982), pp. 1202–10

Cutler, P., 'Contributions to UNICEF/FAO/NPU/ICAR Workshop on Nutrition in Agriculture, Hissar, as follows:

Topic *1c* Current research priorities in nutritional science; *2b* The measurement of poverty: a review of attempts to quantify the poor with special reference to India; *7a* The social effects of agrarian change: the impact of the 'green revolution' in Indian agriculture; *7b* The role of agriculture in economic development in India; *11* The commercialisation of agriculture: trends in agricultural production in India 1891–1978; *11c* Some current arguments on the causes of famine; *4b* Current nutrition planning proposals in India; *13b* Time and income-related changes in supply and consumption patterns of food, 1982a

Cutler, P., 'Blaming underdevelopment on undernutrition'; and 'Some approaches to nutrition project appraisal', in: *Supplementary Reading File*, UNICEF/FAO/NPU/ICAR Workshop on Nutrition and Agriculture, London School of Hygiene and Tropical Medicine, December, 1982b

Dandekar, V.M., 'On measurement of poverty', *Economic and Political Weekly*, **16** (30) (25 July 1981), pp. 1241–50

Dandekar, V.M. and Rath, N., *Poverty in India*, Delhi: Indian School of Political Economy; reprinted from *Economic and Political Weekly* **6** (1 and 2), (2 and 9 January 1971)

Devkota, S., 'Monitoring rural development with nutritional status assessment', MSc thesis, Department of Human Nutrition, London School of Hygiene and Tropical Medicine, 1981

DHSS, *Recommended Intakes of Nutrients for the United Kingdom*, Department of Health and Social Security, Reports on Public Health, no. 120, London: HMSO, 1969

DHSS, *Recommended Daily Amounts of Food Energy and Nutrients for Groups of People in the United Kingdom*, Department of Health and Social Security, London: HMSO, 1979

Dobbins, J. and Widdowson, E.M., 'The effect of undernutrition and subsequent rehabilitation on myelination of rat brain', *Brain*, **88** (1965), p. 357

Doughty, J., 'Dangers of reducing the range of food choice in developing countries', *Ecology of Food and Nutrition*, **8** (1979), pp. 9–12

Dowler, E.A., 'A pilot survey of domestic food wastage', *Journal of Human Nutrition*, **31** (1977), p. 171

Dowler, E.A., Payne, P.R., Seo, Y.O., Thomson, A.M. and Wheeler, E.A., 'Nutrition status indicators: interpretation and policy-making role', *Food Policy*, **7** (1982), pp. 99–112

Dowler, E.A. and Seo, Y.O., 'Assessment of energy intake: supply versus consumption', Contribution to UNICEF/FAO/NPU/ICAR Workshop on Nutrition in Agriculture, Hissar; also *Food Policy* (in press)

Dugdale, A.E. and Payne, P.R., 'Pattern of lean and fat deposition in adults', *Nature* (London), **266** (1977), pp. 349–51

Durkin, N., Ogar, D.A., Tilve, S.G. and Margen, S., 'Human protein requirements: autocorrelation and adaptation to a low protein diet', Joint FAO/WHO/UNU Expert Consultation on Energy and Protein Requirements, 1981

Durnin, J.V.G.A., 'Nutrition (a review)', *Philosophical Transactions of the Royal Society*, **274B** (1976), pp. 447–55

*Dyson, T. and Moore, M., 'On kinship structure, female autonomy, and demographic behaviour in India', *Population and Development Review*, **9** (1983), pp. 35–60

Economic and Political Weekly, 'Levels of Food Consumption', *Economic and Political Weekly* (13 January 1979)

Economist, 'The imperfect 85%' (unsigned), *The Economist* (London), **286** (19 March 1983), p. 54

Epstein, S., *Economic Development and Social Change in South India*, Manchester University Press, 1962

Eusebio, J.S. and Nube, M., 'Attainable growth', letters to the editor, *Lancet*, (28 November 1981), p. 1223

Evans, D.E., Moodie, A.D. and Hansen, J.D.L., 'Kwashiorkor and intellectual development', *South African Medical Journal*, **45** (1971), pp. 1413–26

Eveleth, P.V. and Tanner, J.M., *Worldwide variation in Human Growth*, Cambridge: Cambridge University Press, 1976

*Evenson, R.E., 'Food policy and the new home economics', *Food Policy*, **6** (1981), pp. 180–93

FAO, *World Food Survey*, Washington DC: FAO, 1946

228 *Bibliography*

FAO, *The Second World Food Survey*, Rome: FAO, 1952

FAO, *Calorie Requirements*. Rome: FAO Nutrition Studies, nos. 15 and 16, 1957

FAO, *The Third World Food Survey*, Rome: FAO, 1963

FAO, *Joint FAO/WHO Ad-Hoc Expert Committee Report on Protein and Energy Requirements*, Rome: FAO Nutrition Meetings Report Series, no. 52, 1973

FAO, *Assessment of the World Food Situation*, Rome: FAO, 1974

FAO, *The Fourth World Food Survey*, Rome: FAO Statistics Series, no.11, 1977

FAO, *Food Balance Sheets 1975–77*, Rome: FAO, 1980

FAO, 'Introducing nutrition in agricultural and rural development', Document COAG 81/6, Committee on Agriculture, Sixth Session, Rome: FAO, 1981

FAO, *Integrating Nutrition into Agricultural and Rural Development Projects*, Rome: FAO Nutrition in Agriculture, no. 1, 1983

FAO/WHO, World Health Organisation Technical Report Series, no. 301, Geneva: World Health Organisation, 1965

FAO/WHO, *Requirements of Vitamin A, Thiamine, Riboflavin, and Niacin*, Nutrition Meetings Report Series, no. 41, Geneva: World Health Organisation, 1967

FAO/WHO, *Requirements of Ascorbic Acid, Vitamin D, Vitamin B_{12}, Folate and Iron*, Nutrition Meetings Report Series, no. 47, Geneva: World Health Organisation, 1970

FAO/WHO, *Energy and Protein Requirements*, Geneva: WHO Technical Report Series, no. 522, 1973

*Farmer, B.H. (ed.)., *Green Revolution?*, London and Basingstoke: Macmillan, 1977

Farmer, B.H., 'The "green revolution" in South Asian rice fields: environment and production', *Journal of Development Studies*, 15 (1979), pp. 304–19

Farruk, M.O., 'The structure and performance of the rice marketing system in East Pakistan', Department of Agricultural Economics Occasional Paper no. 3l, Cornell University, Ithaca, New York, 1970

Faulkner, M.D., Reed, G.W. and Brown, D.D., 'Report to the

Government of India on increasing outturns of rice from paddy in India', Intensive Agricultural District Programme, Ford Foundation, Delhi, mimeo, 1963

Fox, R.G., *From Zamindar to Ballot Box*, Ithaca: NY: Cornell University Press, 1969

Fox, R.H., 'A study of energy expenditures of Africans engaged in various rural activities', PhD thesis, University of London, 1953

*Freire, P., *The Pedagogy of the Oppressed*, New York: Seabury Press, 1970

*Freire, P., *Education as the Practice of Freedom*, New York: Seabury Press, 1973

Galbraith, J.K., *The New Industrial State*, (2nd British edn.), London: André Deutsch, 1972

Garza, C., Scrimshaw, N.S. and Young, V.R., 'Human protein requirements: a long-term metabolic study', *Journal of Nutrition,* **107** (1977), pp. 335–52

Geertz, C., *Pedlars and Princes*, Chicago: University of Chicago Press, 1963

George, P.S., *Public Distribution of Foodgrains in Kerala*, Washington: IFPRI Research Report no. 7, 1979

*George, S., *How the Other Half Dies: the Real Reasons for World Hunger*, (revised edn), Harmondsworth: Penguin, 1977

*George, S., *Feeding the Few: Corporate Control of Food*, Washington and Amsterdam: Institute of Policy Studies, 1980

Giama, S.M., 'The relationship between nutritional status and labour productivity', MSc report, Department of Human Nutrition, London School of Hygiene and Tropical Medicine, 1982

Gomez, F., Galvan, R.R., Frank, S., Munoz, J.C., Chavez, R. and Vazquez, R., 'Mortality in second and third degree malnutrition', *Journal of Tropical Pediatrics,* **2** (1956), pp. 77–83

Gopalan, C., 'Observations on some epidemiological factors of protein-calorie malnutrition', in A. van Muralt (ed.), *Protein Calorie Malnutrition*, New York, 1969

Gopalan, C., '"Small is healthy", for the poor not for the rich', *Bulletin of the Nutrition Foundation of India*, (October 1983); also *Economic and Political Weekly,* **18** (15) (1983), p. 591

Government of India, *Annual Report of the Ministry of Food, Cooperation and Community Development*, Delhi: Ministry of Food, 1965

Government of India, *Statistical Abstracts*, Delhi: Central Statistical Office, 1978

Government of India, *A Quick Evaluation of the Food for Work Programme*, Delhi: Planning Commission, Programme Evaluation Organisation, 1980

Government of India, *Sixth Five Year Plan, 1980–85* (prepared 1980, released 1981), Delhi: Planning Commission, 1981

Gracey, M., Cullity, C.J. and Suharjono, S., 'The stomach and malnutrition', *Archives of Diseases in Childhood,* **52** (1977), pp. 325–7

Grande, F., 'Adaptation to environment', in D.B. Hill (ed.), *Handbook of Physiology*, Washington DC: American Physiological Society, 1964

Grantham-McGregor, S., Steward, M.E. and Schofield, W.N., 'Effect of long-term psychological stimulation on mental development of severely malnourished children', *The Lancet*, no. 2 (1980), pp. 785–9

*Greeley, M., 'Appropriate rural technology: recent Indian experience with farm-level foodgrain storage research', *Food Policy,* **3** (1978), pp. 39–49

Guardian, 'Malnutrition threat in India', *Guardian* (Manchester) (29 December 1982)

*Gulati, Leela., *Profiles in Female Poverty: a Study of Five Poor Working Women in Kerala*, New Delhi: Hindustan Publishing Company, and Oxford: Pergamon Press, 1981

Gupta, R.C., *Agricultural Prices in a Backward Economy*, Delhi: National 1973

*Gwatkin, D.R., 'Food policy, nutrition planning, and survival – the cases of Kerala and Sri Lanka', *Food Policy,* **4** (1979), pp. 245–58

*Habicht, J.-P., 'Some characteristics of indicators of nutritional status for use in screening and surveillance', *American*

Journal of Clinical Nutrition, **33** (1980), pp. 531–5

Habicht, J.-P., Martorell, R., Yarborough, C., Malina, R.M. and Klein, R.E., 'Height and weight standards for preschool children. How relevant are ethnic differences in growth potential?', *Lancet, i* (1974), pp. 611–15

Habicht, J.-P., Meyers, L.D. and Brownie, C., 'Indicators for identifying and counting the improperly nourished', *American Journal of Clinical Nutrition*, **35** no.5 (1982), pp. 1241–54

Harriss, B., 'Paddy processing in India and Sri Lanka', *Tropical Science*, **18** (3) (1976), pp. 161–85

Harriss, B., 'Paddy milling: problems in policy and choice of technology', in B.H. Farmer (ed.), *Green Revolution?*, London and Basingtoke: Macmillan, 1977

Harriss, B., *Paddy and Rice Marketing in Northern Tamil Nadu*, Madras: Sangam Publishing Co., 1979

Harriss, B., 'Relevant and feasible research for ICRISAT's Research Program in Agricultural Markets', Progress Report no.6, Economics Program, ICRISAT, Hyderabad, 1980

Harriss, B., Contributions to the UNICEF/FAO/NPU/ICAR Workshop on Nutrition in Agriculture, Hissar, as follows: Topic *6* Stated and implicity priorities in agricultural research; *11a* The process of commercialisation of agricultural commodities in India; *11b* The food marketing system in India; *9b* Theories of the provisioning of the peasant household; *14b* Food distribution, see Harriss (1983c),

Harriss, B., 'Markets and rural undernutrition', London School of Hygiene and Tropical Medicine, mimeo (1983a)

Harriss, B., *Coarse Grains, Coarse Interventions*, Delhi: 21st Century Publishing Trust, 1983b

Harriss, B., 'Implementing food distribution policies: a case study in South India', *Food Policy*, **8** (1983c), pp. 121–30

*Harriss, B., with Chapman, G., McLean, W., Shears, E. and Watson, E., *Exchange Relations and Poverty in Dryland Agriculture*, Delhi: Concept, 1984

Harriss, B. and Kelly, C., 'Policy for rice and oil technology in South Asia', UNICEF/FAO/NPU/ICAR Workshop on Nutrition in Agriculture, Hissar; also in *IDS Bulletin* (Institute of Development Studies, University of Sussex), **13** (3) (1982), pp. 32–45

*Harriss, J., *Capitalism and Peasant Farming*, Bombay: Oxford University Press, 1982

Hertzig, M.E., Birch, H.G., Richardson, S.A. and Tizard, J., 'Intellectual development of school children malnourished during the first years of life', *Pediatrics*, **49** (1972), pp. 812–24

Hicks, N., 'Economic growth and human resources', World Bank Staff Working Paper, no. 403, 1980

Hiernaux, J., 'Weight/height relationship during growth in Africans and Europeans, *Human Biology*, **36** (1964), pp. 273–93

Hildebrand, P.E., 'Combining disciplines in rapid appraisal', *Agricultural Administration*, **8** (6) (1981), pp. 423–32

Horton, S. and King, T., 'Labour productivity', World Bank Staff Working Paper, no. 497, 1981

Howes, M., 'The uses of indigenous technical knowledge in development', *IDS Bulletin* (Institute of Development Studies, University of Sussex), **10** (2) (1979), pp. 12–23

Illich, I., *Limits to Medicine: Medical Nemesis: the Expropriation of Health*, London: Marion Boyars, 1976

Immink, M.D.C., Viteri, F.E. and Helms, R.W., 'Energy intake over the life cycle and human capital formation in Guatemalan sugarcane cutters', *Economic Development and Cultural Change*, **30** (1982), pp. 351–72

IRRI, *Priorities for IRRI's Third Decade*, Los Banos: IRRI, 1982

Ishikawa, S., *Economic Development in Asian Perspective*, Hitosubashi University, Economic Research Series, no.8, Kinokuniya Bookstore Co., Tokyo, 1967

*Jackson, T., *Against the Grain: the Dilemma of Project Food Aid*, Oxford: Oxfam, 1982

Jalil, M.E. and Tahir, W.M., in J.W.G. Porter and B.A. Rolls (eds.), *Proteins in Human Nutrition*, London: Academic Press, 1973

Jazairi, N.T., *Approaches to the Development of Health Indicators*, Paris: OECD Special Studies, no.2, 1976

*Jelliffe, D.B., *The Assessment of the Nutritional Status of the*

Community, Geneva: World Health Organisation, 1966

Jodha, N.S., 'Famine and famine policies: some empirical evidence', *Economic and Political Weekly,* **9** (41) (11 October 1975)

Jones, L., Naughton, J. and Paton, R., *Living with Technology: Block 6, Health* (2nd edn), Milton Keynes: The Open University Press, 1982

Joseph, K., Tasker, P.K., Narayana Rao, M., Swaminathan, M., Sreenivasan, A. and Subrhamanyan, V., 'The effects of supplements of groundnut flour given to undernourished children', *British Journal of Nutrition,* **17** (1963), pp. 13–18

Joy, J.L., 'The economics of food production', *African Affairs,* **65** (1966), p. 261

Joy, J.L., 'Food and nutrition planning theory', in J. Aranda-Pastor and L. Saenz (eds.), *The Process of Food and Nutrition Planning*, Guatemala City: Institute of Nutrition of Central America and Panama (INCAP), 1980

*Joy, J.L. and Payne, P.R., 'Food and nutrition planning', Rome: FAO Consultants' Report Series, no. 35, 1975

Kasongo Project Team, 'Anthropometric assessment of young children's nutritional status as an indicator of subsequent risk of dying', *Journal of Tropical Pediatrics,* **29** (1983), pp. 69–75

Keller, W., Donoso, G. and DeMaeyer, E.M., 'Anthropometry in nutritional surveillance', *Nutrition Abstracts and Reviews,* **46** (1976), pp. 591–609

Kelly, C., 'Oilseeds processing technologies in South India', unpublished MA thesis, School of Development Studies, University of East Anglia, Norwich, 1981

Keys, A., 'Overweight, obesity, coronary heart disease and mortality', *Nutrition Reviews,* **38** (1980), p. 297

Keys, A., Brozek, J., Henschell, A., Mickelson, O. and Taylor, H.L., *The Biology of Human Starvation*, (2 vols.), Minneapolis: University of Minnesota Press, 1950

Khan, M.U., 'Breastfeeding, growth and diarrhoea in rural Bangladesh children', *Human Nutrition: Clinical Nutrition,* **38C** (1984), pp. 113–19

Khare, B.P., 'Insect pests of stored grain and their control in Uttar Pradesh'. G.B. Pant University of Agriculture and

Technology, Pan nagar, Naindal UP, 1972

Kielmann, A.A. and McCord, C., 'Weight-for-age as an index of risk of death in children', *The Lancet*, no.1 (1978), pp. 1247–50

Kirkwood, T.B.L., 'The evolution of ageing', *Nature* (London) **270** (1977), p. 301

Kleiber, M., *The Fire of Life: an Introduction to Animal Energetics*, New York: Wiley, 1961

Kleitman, N., 'Basal metabolism in prolonged fasting in man', *American Journal of Physiology*, **77** (1926), pp. 233–44

Krishnaji, R., 'Wheat price movements: an analysis', *Economic and Political Weekly*, **8** (26) (1973)

Krishnaji, R., 'State intervention in foodgrains prices', *Social Scientist*, no. 31 (1975), pp. 75–90

Krishnamurthy, J., 'Working force in 1971: unilluminating final results', *Economic and Political Weekly*, special no. (August 1973), pp. 31–3

Kuhn, T.S., *The Structure of Scientific Revolutions* (2nd edn), Chicago: University of Chicago Press, 1970

Kumar, D., 'Changes in income distribution and poverty in India', *World Development*, **2** (1973), p. 35, table 4

Kurien, P.P., Swaminathan, M. and Subrhamanyan, V., *Journal of Food Science*, **11** (1961), p. 214

Laar, A. van der, *The World Bank and the Poor*, Boston and London: Martinus Nijhoff Publications, 1980

Lal, D., 'Agricultural growth: real wages and the rural poor', *Economic and Political Weekly*, **11** (26) (1976), pp. A47–A61

Latham, M.C., 'Protein-calorie malnutrition in children and its relation to psychological development and behaviour', *Physiological Reviews*, **54** (1974), pp. 541–55

Latham, M.C., Stephenson, L.S., Hall, A., Wolgemuth, J.C., Elliot, T.C. and Crompton, D.W.T., 'Parasitic infections, anaemia and nutritional status: a study of their interrelationships and the effect of prophylaxis and treatment on workers in Kwale District, Kenya', *Transactions of the Royal Society of Tropical Medicine and Hygiene*, **77** (1) (1983), pp. 41–8

Leach, G., 'Energy and food production', *Food Policy*, **1** (1975) pp. 62–73

Lele, U.J., *Modernisation of the rice industry* (reprinted from *Economic and Political Weekly*), Ithaca, NY: Department of Agricultural Economics, Cornell University, 1970

Lele, U.J., *Foodgrain Marketing in India*, Ithaca, NY: Cornell University Press, 1971

*Levinson, J.F., *Morinda: an Economic Analysis of Malnutrition among Young Children in rural India*, Cambridge, Mass.: MIT Press, 1974

Liebenstein, H., *Economic Backwardness and Economic Growth*, New York: Wiley, 1957

*Lipton, M. *Poverty, Undernutrition and Hunger*, World Bank Staff Working Paper, no. 597, 1982

Lipton, M., *Labor and Poverty*, World Bank Staff Working Paper, no. 616, 1983

Longhurst, R. and Payne, P., *Seasonal Aspects of Nutrition: Review of Evidence and Policy Implications*, Institute of Development Studies, University of Sussex, discussion paper 145, 1979

Lowe, M., 'Influence of changing lifestyles' in M. Turner (ed.), *Nutrition and Lifestyles*, London: Applied Science Publishers, 1980

Lunn, P.C., Whitehead, R.G. and Coward, W.A., 'Two pathways to kwashiorkor?', *Transactions of the Royal Society of Tropical Medicine and Hygiene,* **73** (4) (1979), pp. 438–44

McCance, R.A. and Widdowson, E.M., *Calorie Deficiencies and Protein Deficiencies*, London: Churchill, 1968

McIntire, J. and Matlon, P., 'Priorities for ICRISAT's village-level studies program', Draft Research Report, ICRISAT, Ouagadougou, 1981

McKeown, T., *The Role of Medicine*, Oxford: Blackwell, 1979

McLean, W., 'Child Nutrition in Nepal', Report to Save the Children Fund and ODA, 1981

MAFF, *Household Food Consumption and Expenditure 1978*, Annual Report of the National Food Survey Committee, London: HMSO, 1980

Malawi Ministry of Agriculture, *A Guild to the Safe Storage of Cereals, Oilseeds and Pulses,* Lilongwe (Malawi): Extension Aid Branch, 1973

Marr, J., 'Individual dietary surveys: purposes and methods', *World Review of Nutrition and Dietetics,* **13** (1971), pp. 105–61

Martorell, J., Leslie, J. and Moock, P.R., 'Characteristics and determinations of child nutritional status in Nepal', *American Journal of Clinical Nutrition,* **39** (1984), pp. 74–86

Martorell, R., Yarbrough, C., Yarbrough, S. and Klein, R.E., 'The impact of ordinary illnesses on the dietary intakes of malnourished children, *American Journal of Clinical Nutrition,* **33** (1980), pp. 345–50

Mata, L.J., Kromal, R.A., Urrutia, J.J. and Garcia, B., 'Effect of infection on food intake and the nutritional state: perspectives as viewed from the village', *American Journal of Clinical Nutrition,* **30** (1977), pp. 1215–27

Mellor, J.W., *The New Economics of Growth*, Ithaca, NY: Cornell University Press, 1976

Miller, D.S., *The Regulation of Energy Balance in Man*, Geneva: WHO Medicine and Hygiene, 1975

Miller, D.S., 'Man's demand for energy', in K.L. Blaxter (ed.), *Food Chains and Human Nutrition*, Applied Science Publishers, 1979

Miller, D.S. and Mumford, D., 'Gluttony 1: an experimental study of over-eating on high protein diets', *American Journal of Clinical Nutrition,* **20** (1967), p.1212

Miller, D.S. and Rivers, J.P.W., 'Seasonal variations in food intake in two Ethiopian villages', *Proceedings of the Nutrition Society,* **31** (1972), pp. 32–3A

Mishra, S.C., 'Patterns of long-run agrarian change in Bombay and Punjab', unpublished PhD thesis, 1981

Mitchell, H.H., *The Comparative Nutrition of Man and Domestic Animals*, (2 vols.), New York: Academic Press, 1962

Mody, A., 'Growth, distribution and evolution of agricultural markets', *Economic and Political Weekly,* **17** (1, 2) (1982), pp. 25–37

Myrdal, G., *Economic Theory and Underdeveloped Regions*, London: Methuen, 1972

Nabarro, D., 'Social, economic, health and environmental

determinants of nutritional status', *Proceedings of the WHO Workshop on Nutrition Monitoring and Evaluation*, D. Nabarro and A. Pradilla (eds.), Delhi: WHO, 1981

Nabarro, D., 'The domestic environment: food, fuel and diarrhoea', Paper presented at the UNICEF/FAO/NPU/ICAR Workshop on Nutrition in Agriculture, Hissar, 1982

*Nadkarni, M.V., 'Marketable surplus, market dependence and economic development', *Social Scientist,* **83** (1979), pp. 35–50

Nanda, J.S. and Coffman, W.F., 'IRRI's efforts to improve the protein content of rice', in *Chemical Aspects of Rice Grain Quality* (workshop proceedings), Los Banos (Philippines): IRRI, 1979

NAS, *Recommended Dietary Allowances*, Washington DC: National Academy of Sciences, 1943

NAS, ibid. (2nd edn), 1945

NAS, ibid. (3rd edn), 1948

NAS, ibid. (5th edn), 1958

NAS, ibid. (6th edn), 1963

NAS, ibid. (7th edn), 1968

NAS, ibid. (8th edn), 1974

NCDC, *Chandigarh Seminar Proceedings*, Delhi: National Cooperative Development Corporation, 1975

NCDC, *Workshop on Cooperative Oilseed Processing Industry*, background paper, 28–29 January, Delhi: National Cooperative Development Corporation, 1980

Nepal Children's Organisation, 'Dhankuta Project Report', Kathmandu: NCO 1980

Ngoddy, P.O., 'Gari mechanisation in Nigeria', in N. Jequier (ed.) *Appropriate Technology: Problems and Promises*, Paris: OECD Development Centre, 1976

Nicol, B.M. and Phillips, P.G., 'Endogenous nitrogen excretion and utilisation of dietary protein', *British Journal of Nutrition,* **35** (1976), p. 181

Norgan, N.G., Ferro-Luzzi, A. and Durnin, J.V.G.A., 'The energy and nutrient intake of 204 New Guinea adults', *Philosophical Transactions of the Royal Society,* **268B** (1974) pp. 309–48

NRC, *World Food and Nutrition Study: the Potential Contributions of Research*, Washington DC: National Research Council, National Academy of Sciences, 1977

Ojha, P.O., 'A configuration of India poverty', *Reserve Bank of India Bulletin* (January, 1970)

Omawale, 'Nutrition protein identification and development policy implications, *Ecology of Food and Nutrition*, **9** (1980), pp. 113–22

Oomen, H.A.P.C., McLaren, D.S. and Escapini, H., 'Epidemiology and public health aspects of hypovitaminosis A', *Tropical and Geographical Medicine*, **4** (1974), p. 271

Oppen, M. von, 'Consumer preferences for quality characters of dryland food crops', Economics Program Report, ICRISAT, Hyderabad, 1979

Orr, J.B., *Food, Health and Income*, London: Macmillan, 1936

Orr, J.B., *As I Recall*, London: MacGibbon and Kee, 1966

Pacey, A., *Gardening for Better Nutrition*, London: Intermediate Technology Publications, 1978

Pacey, A., *The Culture of Technology*, Oxford: Blackwell, and Cambridge, Mass.: MIT Press, 1983

Padfield, N. and Nabarro, D., 'Vitamin A deficiency in Dhankuta', *Journal of the Institute of Medicine of Nepal*, **2** (1981), pp. 147–60

Pain, A., 'Nutritional criteria in plant breeding', paper presented to the UNICEF/FAO/NPU/ICAR Workshop on Nutrition in Agriculture, Hissar, 1982

Palmer, I., 'The new rice in Indonesia', in I. Palmer (ed.), *The New Rice in Asia: Conclusions from Four Country Studies*, Geneva: UNRISD, 1972

Parpia, H.A.B. and Desikachar, H.S.R., 'Modern process for parboiling rice', in *Modernisation in Rice Industry*, Ahmedabad: Indian Institute of Management, 1969, pp. 83–8

Paul, A.A., Muller, E.M. and Whitehead, R.G., 'The quantitative effects of maternal dietary energy intake on pregnancy and lactation in rural Gambian women', *Transactions of the Royal Society of Tropical Medicine and Hygiene*, **73** (6) (1979), pp. 686–92

Payne, P.R., 'Protein quality of diets, chemical scores and amino acid imbalances', *International Encyclopaedia of Food and Nutrition*, Vol. II (1972)

Payne, P.R., 'Safe protein-calorie ratios in diets', *American Journal of Clinical Nutrition*, 28 (1975), pp. 281–6

Payne, P.R., 'Nutritional criteria for breeding and selection of crops', *Plant Foods for Man*, 2 (1976), pp. 95–112

Payne, P.R., Contributions to UNICEF/FAO/NPU/ICAR Workshop on Nutrition in Agriculture, Hissar, as follows: Topic *1* Variability of nutrient requirements; *1c* Human nutrition and agricultural development: past and present perspectives; *9a* Nutrient and energy requirements and the agrarian ecology; *13* Nutritional criteria for influencing national food policies, 1982

Payne, P.R. and Dugdale, A.E., 'A model for the prediction of energy balance and body weight', *Annals of Human Biology*, 4 (6) (1977), pp. 525–35

*Pearse, A., *Seeds of Plenty, Seeds of Want: Social and Economic Implications of New Varieties of Foodgrains*, Oxford: Clarendon Press, 1981

Pearse, A. (ed.), *The Social and Economic Implications of Large-scale Introduction of New Varieties of Foodgrain*, see UNRISD, 1974

Penemangalore, M., Parthasarathy, H.N., Joseph, K., Narayana Rao, M., Indiramma, K., Rajagopalan, R., Swaminathan, M., Screenivasan, A. and Subrahmanyan, V., *Journal of Food Science*, 11 (1962), p. 214

Pereira, S.M., Jones, S., Jesudian, G. and Begum, A., 'Feeding trials with lysine and threonine fortified rice', *British Journal of Nutrition*, 30 (1973), pp. 241–50

Pingle, V., 'Some studies in two tribal groups of central India', *Plant Foods for Man*, 1 (1975), p. 185

Poleman, T.T., 'A reappraisal of the extent of world hunger', *Food Policy*, 6 (1981), pp. 236–52

Popper, K.R., *The Open Society and its Enemies* (2 vols; the passage quoted is in vol.1, notes for ch. 9), London: Routledge, 1945

Praun, A., 'Nutrition education: development or alienation?',

Human Nutrition: Applied Nutrition, **36A** (1982), pp. 28–34

Prentice, A.M., Whitehead, R.G., Roberts, S.B. and Paul, A.A., 'Long-term energy balance in child-bearing Gambian women', *American Journal of Clinical Nutrition,* **34** (1981), pp. 2790–9

Raj, K.N., 'Peasants and potatoes', *Mainstreams,* **19** (23) (1981), pp. 4–6

Rao, V.B., 'Measurement of deprivation and poverty', *World Development,* **9** (4) (1981)

Rao, V.K.R.V., 'Nutritional norms by calorie intake and measurement of poverty', *Bulletin of the International Statistical Institute,* 41st Session, **43**, Book 1 (1977), pp. 645–54

Rao, V.K.R.V., 'Measurement of poverty: a note', *Economic and Political Weekly,* **16** (35) (29 August 1981)

Reddy, V., Jagadeesan, N., Ragharamulu, C., Bhaskaram, C. and Srikantia, S.G., 'Functional significance of growth retardation in malnutrition', *American Journal of Clinical Nutrition,* **29** (1976), pp. 3–7

Reeds, P.J., Fuller, M.F., Cadenhead, A., Lobley, G.B. and McDonald, J.D., 'Effects of changes in the intake of protein in growing pigs', *British Journal of Nutrition,* **45** (1981), pp. 539–46

Reutlinger, S. and Alderman, H., 'Prevalence of calorie deficient diets in developing countries', World Bank Staff Working Paper, no. 374, 1980

Reutlinger, S. and Selowsky, M., *Malnutrition and Poverty,* Baltimore: Johns Hopkins University Press, 1976

Richards, P., 'Community environmental knowledge in African rural development', *IDS Bulletin* (Institute of Development Studies, University of Sussex), **10**, (2) (1979), p. 28

Richards, P., 'Appraising appraisal: towards improved dialogue in rural planning', *IDS Bulletin* (Institute of Development Studies, University of Sussex) **12** (4) (1981), pp. 8–11

Richards, P., '"Participatory" research in rural development', Contribution to UNICEF/FAO/NPU/ICAR Workshop on Nutrition and Agriculture, Hissar, 1982

Rickleton, J., 'Nutrition and agriculture in East Nepal', MSc thesis, Department of Human Nutrition, London School of

Hygiene and Tropical Medicine, 1981

*Rivers, J.P.W. and Payne, P.R., 'The comparison of energy supply and energy need: a critique of energy requirements', in: G.A. Harrison (ed.), *Energy and Effort* (Proceedings of a symposium), London: Taylor and Francis, 1982

Roberts, N.C.E., 'Programmes and studies', MPhil thesis, University of Reading, Department of Agricultural Economics, 1981

Roberts, S.B., Paul, A.A., Cole, T.J. and Whitehead, R.G., 'Seasonal changes in activity, birthweight and lactational performance in rural Gambian women', *Transactions of the Royal Society of Hygiene and Tropical Medicine*, **76** (5) (1982), pp. 668–78

Rogers, E.M., *Modernisation among Peasants*, New York: Holt, Rinehart and Winston, 1969

Ross, M.H., Lustbader, E. and Bras, G., 'Dietary practices and growth responses as predictors of longevity', *Nature,* **262** (1976), p. 548

Rowland, M., 'The diarrhoea-malnutrition complex', *Diarrhoea Dialogue*, no. 6, (August 1984), p. 4; also editorial, p. 1

Rowland, M.G.M., Barrell, R.A.E. and Whitehead, R.G., 'Bacterial contamination in traditional Gambian weaning foods', *The Lancet*, no. 1 (1978), pp. 136–8

Rowland, M.G.M., Paul, A., Prentice, A.M., Miller, E., Hutton, M., Barrell, R.A.E. and Whitehead, R.G., 'Seasonality and the growth of infants in a Gambian village', in: R. Chambers, R. Longhurst and A. Pacey (eds.), *Seasonal Dimensions to Rural Poverty*, London: Francis Pinter, 1981

Rowntree, B.S., *Poverty: a Study of Town Life*, London: Macmillan, 1901

Rudra, A., 'The organisation of agriculture for rural development', *Cambridge Journal of Economics,* **2** (1978), pp. 381–406

Rutishauser, I.H.E., 'Factors affecting the intake of energy and protein by Ugandan preschool children', *Ecology of Food and Nutrition,* **3** (1974), p. 213

Ruttan, V., 'Institutional factors affecting the generation and diffusion of agricultural technology', World Employment

Programme Research Working Paper, WEP 2/-22/WP67, Geneva: International Labour Office, 1980

Ryan, J., Sheldrake, G.R. and Yadav, S.P., 'Human nutritional needs and crop breeding objectives in the semi-arid tropics', Occasional Paper no. 4, Economics Program, ICRISAT, Hyderabad, 1974

Ryle, J.A., *Changing Disciplines*, London: Oxford University Press, 1948

Sarma, J.A. and Roy, S., 'Behaviour of foodgrain production and consumption in India, 1960–77', World Bank Staff Working Paper, no. 339, 1979

Satyanarayana, K., Nadamuni Naidu, A., Chatterjee, B., and Narasingha Rao, B.S., 'Body size and work output', *American Journal of Clinical Nutrition*, **30** (1977), pp.322–5

*Schaffer, B., and Lamb, G.B., *Can Equity be Organised?*, Farnborough: Gower, 1981

Schapera, I., *Married Life in an African Tribe*, Harmondsworth: Penguin (original edition was 1940), 1971

Schofield, S., 'Seasonal factors affecting nutrition in different age groups', *Journal of Development Studies*, **11** (1974), pp. 22–40

*Schofield, S., *Development and the Problems of Village Nutrition*, London: Croom Helm, 1979

Schultz, T.W., *Transforming Traditional Agriculture*, New Haven, Conn.: Yale University Press, 1964

Scott, W. and Mathew, N.T., *A Development Monitoring Service at the Local Level: Volume 2, Levels of Living and Poverty in Kerala*, Geneva: UNRISD, 1983

*Seaman, J., and Holt, J., 'Markets and famines in the Third World', *Disasters*, **4** (1980), pp. 283–97

Seckler, D., 'Optimal body size and a possible production constant', Ford Foundation, New Delhi, mimeo, 1981

Selowsky, M., and Taylor, L., 'The economics of malnourished children', *Economic Development and Cultural Change*, **22** (1) (1970), pp. 17–30

Sen, A. K., 'Poverty, inequality and unemployment', in T.N. Srinivasan and P.K. Bardhan (eds.), *Poverty and Income*

Distribution in India, Calcutta: Statistical Publishing Society, 1974

*Sen, A.K., *Poverty and Famines*, Oxford: Oxford University Press, 1981

Sen, A.K., Book reviews, *Journal of Peasant Studies,* **10** (4) (1983), pp. 274–5

Sen, A.K. and Senqupta, S., 'Malnutrition of rural children and the sex bias', *Economic and Political weekly*, Annual number (May 1983), pp. 855–64

Seo, Y.O., 'The pattern of nutrition indicators at different stages of national development', PhD thesis, University of London, Faculty of Medicine 1981

Sewell, W.R.D., 'The role of perception of professionals in environmental decision-making', in A. Porteous, K. Attenborough and C. Pollit (eds.), *Pollution: the Professionals and the Public*, Milton Keynes: Open University Press, 1977

Sheldon, E. and Moore, W.E., *Indicators of Social Change*, New York: Russell Sage Foundation, 1968

Shetty, S.L., 'Structural retrogression in the economy', *Economic and Political Weekly,* **12** (6–7) (1978)

Simmons, E.B., 'The small-scale rural food processing industry in Northern Nigeria', *Food Research Institute Studies*, (Stanford), **14** (2) (1975), pp. 147–62

Singh, S.P., *Centre-State Relations in Agriculture Development*, Delhi: Vikas, 1973

Smith, P. and Hagard, S., 'Planning for a single speciality in a health district', *Journal of the Operational Research Society,* **33** (1982), pp. 29–39

Sopher, D.E. (ed.), *An Exploration of India*, London: Longman, and Ithaca, NY: Cornell University Press, 1980

Spence, J., *The Purpose and Practice of Medicine*, London: Oxford University Press, 1960

Spitz, P., *Food Systems and Society in India*, Geneva: UNRISD, 1983

*Srinivasan, T.N., 'Trends in agriculture in India, 1949–50 to 1977–78', *Economic and Political Weekly,* **14** (special number) (August 1979)

Stein, Z., Susser, M., Saenger, G., and Marolla, F., 'Nutrition and mental performance', *Science,* **173** (1972), pp. 708–13

Stevens, C., *Food Aid and the Developing World*, London: Croom Helm in association with Overseas Development Institute, 1979

Stoch, M.B. and Smythe, P.M., 'Does undernutrition during infancy inhibit brain growth?', *Archives of Disease in Childhood,* **38** (1963), pp. 546–51

*Sukhatme, P.V., 'The world's hunger and future needs in food supplies', *Journal of the Royal Statistical Society,* A., **124** (1961), pp. 463–525

Sukhatme, P.V., 'Measuring the incidence of undernutrition: a comment', *Economic and Political Weekly,* **16** (23) (6 June 1981a)

Sukhatme, P.V., 'On measurement of poverty', *Economic and Political Weekly,* **16** (32) (8 August 1981b), pp. 1323–4

Sukhatme, P.V., 'Relationship between malnutrition and poverty', First National Conference on Social Science, January 1981, Delhi: National Council of Applied Economic Research, mimeo, 1981c

*Sukhatme, P.V., and Margen, S., 'Models for protein deficiency', *American Journal of Cinical Nutrition,* **31** (1978), p. 1237

Swaminathan, M.C., 'National Nutrition Monitoring Bureau in India', Contribution to the UNICEF/FAO/NPU/ICAR Workshop on Nutrition in Agriculture, Hissar 1982

Talbot, F.B., 'Measurement of obesity by the creatinine coefficient', *American Journal of Diseases of Childhood,* **55** (1938), p. 455

Tandon, B.N., Ramachandran, K., and Gupta, M.C., 'Effect of health and nutrition status of road construction workers in Northern India on productivity', World Bank Technical Memorandum, no. 4, Washington, 1975

Tasker, P.K., Doraiswamy, T.R., Narayanarao, M., Swaminathan, M., Sreenivasan, A., and Subrahmanyan, V., 'The metabolism of nitrogen, calcium and phosphorus in undernourished children', *British Journal of Nutrition,* **16** (1962), pp. 361–8

Thakur, D.S., 'Food grain marketing efficiency', *Indian*

Journal of Agricultural Economics, **29** (4) (1974), pp. 61–5

Timmer, C.P., 'A model of rice marketing margins in Indonesia', *Food Research Institute Studies* (Stanford), **13** (2) (1974), pp. 145–67

Tizard, J., 'Ecological studies of malnutrition', University of London, Institute of Education, mimeo, 1973

Tomkins, A.M., 'Nutritional status and severity of diarrhoea among preschool children in rural Nigeria', *The Lancet*, no. 1 (1981), pp. 560–2

Tomkins, A.M., 'Nutritional cost of protracted diarrhoea in young Gambian children', *GUT,* **24** (1983), A 459

Tonon, M., 'Models for educational intervention in malnourished populations', *American Journal of Clinical Nutrition,* **31** (1978), pp. 2279–83

Trowbridge, F.L., 'Anthropometric criteria in malnutrition', *The Lancet,* no. 2 (1979), pp. 589–90

Trowbridge, F.L. and Staehling, N., 'Sensitivity and specificity of arm circumference indicators in identifying malnourished children', *American Journal of Clinical Nutrition,* **33** (3) (1980), pp. 687–96

United Nations, *Poverty, Unemployment and Development Policy*, Geneva: United Nations, 1975

*UNRISD, *The Social and Economic Implications of Large-scale Introduction of New Varieties of Foodgrain*, A. Pearse (ed.), Geneva: United Nations Research Institute for Social Development, 1974

USDA, *World Food Budget, 1962 and 1966*, Washington DC: United States Department of Agriculture, 1961

USDA, *World Food Budget 1970*, Washington DC: United States Department of Agriculture, 1964

Valverde, V., Martorell, R., Meija Pivaral, V., Delgado, H., Lechtig, A., Teller, C. and Klein, R.E., 'Relationship between family land availability and nutritional status', *Ecology of Food and Nutrition,* **6** (1977), pp. 1–7

Valverde, V., Rojas Z., Vinocur, P., Payne, P. and Thomson, A., 'Organization of an information system for food and nutrition programmes in Costa Rica', **7** (1981b), pp. 32–40

Valverde, V., Vargas, W., Payne, P. and Thomson A., 'Data

requirements and nutrition planning in Costa Rica', *Food Policy,* **6** (1981), pp. 19–26

Walker, C.L. and Church, M., 'Poverty by administration: a review of supplementary benefits, nutrition and scale rate', *Journal of Human Nutrition,* **32** (1978), pp. 5–18

Waterlow, J.C., 'Classification and definition of protein-calorie malnutrition', *British Medical Journal,* no. 3 (1972), pp. 566–9

Waterlow, J.C., 'Classification and definition of protein-energy malnutrition', in *Nutrition in Preventive Medicine,* Geneva: WHO, Annex 5, 1976, pp. 530–55

Waterlow, J.C., 'Adaptation to different intakes and environments', Joint FAO/WHO/UNU Consultation on Energy and Protein Requirements, October 1981

*Waterlow, J.C. and Payne, P.R., 'The protein gap', *Nature* (London), **258** (1975), pp. 113–17

Waterlow, J.C., Ashworth, A. and Griffiths, M., 'Faltering in infant growth in less developed countries', *The Lancet,* no. 2 (1980), pp. 1176–80

Waterlow, J.C. and Rutishauser, I.H.E., in J. Cravioto, L. Hambraeuse and B. Valquist (eds.), *Early Malnutrition and Mental Development,* Stockholm: Almqvist and Wiksell, 1974

Webster, C., 'Healthy or hungry thirties?', *History Workshop Journal,* no. 13 (1983), pp. 110–29

Wenlock, R.W. and Buss, D.H., 'Wastage of edible food in the home', *Journal of Human Nutrition,* **31** (1977), p. 405

Wenlock, R.W., Buss, D.H., Derry, B.J. and Dixon, E.J., 'Household food wastage in Britain', *British Journal of Nutrition,* **43** (1980), p. 53

Wheeler, D., 'Human resource development and economic growth in developing countries: a simulation model', World Bank Staff Working Paper, no. 407, 1980

Wheeler, E.F., Contribution to UNICEF/FAO/NPU/ICAR Workshop on Nutrition in Agriculture, Hissar, as follows: Topic *1b* Themes in nutrition training and research; *9b* Nutritional criteria in provisioning at the household level; *13* Behavioural and cultural determinants of food demand; *14c*

Targeted feeding schemes, 1982

Wheeler, E.F. and Tan, S.P., 'From concept to practice: food behaviour of Chinese immigrants in London', *Ecology of Food and Nutrition*, **13** (1983), pp. 51–7

White, B.N.F., 'Rural household studies in anthropological perspective', in H.P. Binswanger (ed.), *Rural Household Studies in Asia*, Singapore: Singapore University Press, 1980

Whitehead, R.G., 'Infection and the development of kwashiorkor and marasmus in Africa', *American Journal of Clinical Nutrition*, **30** (1977), pp. 1281–4

WHO, *The Assessment of Nutritional Impact*, Geneva: World Health Organisation, 1979

Wija, A., 'The nutritional impact of food-for-work programmes', Report to ODA, London School of Hygiene and Tropical Medicine, 1982a

Wija, A., 'Feeding, illness and nutritional status of children in rural Gujarat', MSc report, London School of Hygiene and Tropical Medicine, 1982b

Williams, C.D., 'A nutritional disease of children associated with maize diet', *Archives of Diseases in Childhood*, **8** (1982b), pp. 423,434

Willson, H.F., 'Rural wheat storage in Ludhiana District', Delhi: Ford Foundation Staff Document, 1970

Winnick, M. and Noble, A., 'Cellular response in rats during malnutrition at various ages', *Journal of Nutrition*, **89** (1966), pp. 300–4

Winnick, M. and Rosso, P., 'Head circumference and cellular growth of the brain in normal and marasmic children', *Journal of Pediatrics*, **74** (1969a), pp. 774–8

Winnick, M. and Rosso., P., 'The effect of severe early malnutrition on cellular growth of the human brain', *Pediatric Research*, **3** (1969b), pp. 181–4

Wood, T.B. and Capstick, J.W., 'The energy requirements of animals', *Journal of Agricultural Science*, **18** (1928), p. 486

Woolf, B., 'Poverty lines and standards of living', *Proceedings of the Nutrition Society*, **5** (1946), pp. 71–81

World Bank, *Malnutrition and Poverty* S. Reutlinger and M. Selowsky (eds.), Baltimore: Johns Hopkins University Press,

1976

World Bank, *World Tables* (2nd edn), Baltimore: Johns Hopkins University Press, 1980

Yoshimura, H., 'Physiological effects of protein deficiency with special reference to evaluation of protein nutrition and protein requirement', *World Review of Nutrition and Dietetics,* **14** (1972), p. 100

Young, K., Wolkowitz, C. and McCullagh, R., *Of Marriage and the Market*, London: CSE Books, 1981

Author index

Numbers in italics refer to figures and tables.

Subject Index

252   *Subject Index*

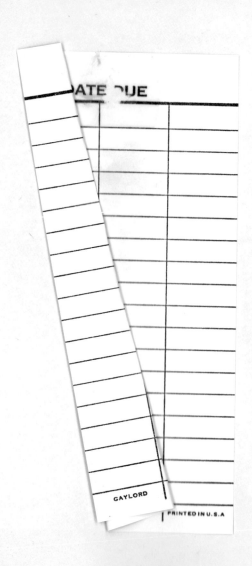

DATE DUE

GAYLORD

PRINTED IN U.S.A